Language, Aphasia, and the Right Hemisphere

Language, Aphasia, and the Right Hemisphere

CHRIS CODE
Leicester Polytechnic

JOHN WILEY & SONS

Chichester · New York · Brisbane · Toronto · Singapore

Library of Congress Cataloging in Publication Data:

Code, Christopher.
  Language, aphasia, and the right Hemisphere.
  Includes index.
  1. Aphasia. 2. Cerebral hemispheres. 3. Cerebral
dominance. 4. Neurolinguistics. I. Title.
RC425.C59   1987   616.85′52   86-15747

ISBN 0 471 91158 5

British Library Cataloguing in Publication Data:

Code, Christopher
  Language, aphasia and the right hemisphere.
  1. Neurolinguistics
  I. Title
  612′.8   QP399
  ISBN 0 471 91158 5

Typeset by Acorn Bookwork, Salisbury, Wiltshire
Printed and bound in Great Britain

DEDICATION

For M. K. Code and Leah Lucas, who like to see their names in print, and for Gabby and Billy, who couldn't care less.

CONTENTS

PREFACE

In little more than a decade our understanding of the role of the right cerebral hemisphere in behaviour in general, and language in particular, has been revolutionized. In that time we have moved from a position where the right hemisphere was seen as a mute, 'word deaf, word blind' and vaguely 'visuo-spatial' processor, to one where it can be seen as a sophisticated neurocognitive processor working in some kind of complementary relationship with the processing responsibilities of the left hemisphere. This area of research is a developing and controversial one, and is likely to remain so for some time yet. While keeping in mind the immaturities of this exciting field, I have tried to present a critical synthesis, with discussion of what I have seen to be the central issues for the present and for developments in the near future, as well as a comprehensive source book.

A few points on the organization of the book may be useful here. Chapter 2 aims to discuss the major methodological problems in neurolinguistic research in a single chapter. Readers who are aware of the limitations of various research methods and the problems of interpretation of much neuro-psychological data may feel no need to read this chapter. Throughout the rest of the book, however, little detailed reference is made to such issues of method and interpretation, and an awareness of the problems is assumed. Although Chapter 3 and 4 are respectively concerned with the right hemisphere's role in linguistic comprehension and expression, this is a pragmatic division of labour which is not meant to imply either psychological or biological division. While early chapters take a broader approach to the research, in Chapter 6, 7, and 8 discussion narrows down to a consideration of the relevance of aphasia to right hemisphere language research and the applications of this research to our understanding of the recovery and rehabilitation of aphasia.

This book should be of relevance to all those with an academic or clinical interest in language–brain relationships: graduates, teachers, researchers and clinicians in neuropsychology, cognitive psychology and clinical psychology, in psycholinguistics and neurolinguistics, and in speech and language pathology and therapy.

I am indebted to a number of friends and colleagues for critical reviews of various parts of this book. Specifically (and alphabetically) I am grateful to Andrew Burton, Andrew Ellis, Guido Gainotti, Yvan Lebrun, John Marshall, Dave Muller, and Harry Purser. Of course, the ideas expressed, and the errors made, are all mine. I also want to thank Edoc Legin for help with illustrations and Danuta Hayward for typing drafts of some of the chapters. Mainly, I want to thank my wife, Chris, for her understanding and her macaroni cheese.

Chris Code
Leicester: April 1986

Chapter One

FROM CEREBRAL DOMINANCE TO COMPLEMENTARY SPECIALIZATION

The neocortex of the human brain is made up of two hemispheres. Since the middle and late 1800s, when Dax (1836, but not published until 1865), Broca (1861, 1865), and Wernicke (1874) first described the language problems that resulted following damage to the left hemisphere, and up until relatively recently, the overwhelming belief was that the relationship between the two cerebral hemispheres was one of dominance by the left and subservience of the right. This 'dominance' notion of a major or superior and a minor or inferior hemisphere, where overriding control of cognitive processing resides in one, owes most to the dogma that the left hemisphere is superior in its ability to process language.

The notion of cerebral dominance has been variously explained, but 'consciousness' itself is central to most explanations. The problem is that there exists a variety of conceptions of the nature of human consciousness, ranging from the relatively simple state of wakefulness, to self-awareness, or some cognitive information-processing system (see Oakley, 1985, for a recent and useful collection on the topic of brain and consciousness). Some of these conceptualizations have been equated with the notion of cerebral (left hemisphere) dominance. Dominance has been characterized as an aspect of 'self-consciousness' (Eccles, 1965, 1973, 1977; Popper and Eccles, 1977), where self-consciousness is seen to be a property primarily of the left hemisphere. Gazzaniga (1974a) sees left hemisphere dominance as a:

> decision processing system ... that is responsible for bringing order to our various mental activities to the final cognitive path. In this view, the term cerebral dominance would refer to the central system that institutes order in a chaotic cognitive space (pp. 367–8).

Gazzaniga suggests, however, that this decision-processing system is superordinate and independent of natural language *per se*. More recently, Gazzaniga (1983) has extended this conceptualization of dominance to include our sense of subjective awareness that:

> arises out of our dominant left hemisphere's unrelenting need to explain actions taken from any one of a multitude of mental systems that dwell within us (p. 536).

Despite the well-documented abilities of the right hemisphere, Gazzaniga suggests that it lacks the kind of cognitive sophistication associated with

1

formal linguistic operations and that the completion of even simple perceptual matching tasks is often lacking from a right hemisphere without linguistic skills. He argues, in fact, that the cognitive skills of the *separated* right hemisphere without linguistic skills (the importance of defining the source of evidence for hemispheric abilities is discussed fully in Chapter 2) are probably inferior to those of a chimpanzee. He concludes that:

> the price of lateral specialization for language on the left is a state of rudimentary cognition for the right hemisphere, which is revealed only if the latter has to serve alone following brain bisection or left-brain damage (1983, p. 536).

Nottebohm (1983) also implies that the notion of left hemisphere dominance is synonymous with decision making when he suggests that 'control of the commencement of behaviour and decision making might be inefficient under equipotential and simultaneous bilateral representation' (p. 75).

Bever (1983) has also suggested, on the basis of a cognitive model of consciousness, that the left hemisphere is 'the seat of consciousness'. He outlines a modular theory of cognition which involves relational (analytic) and unitary (holistic) processing, where, for example, the planned production of a whole syllable will be unitary but the planned production of the syllable as a sequence of separate phonetic segments is relational. On this appreciation, analytic processing is a special form of relational processing, where the relation is between part and whole. Consciousness essentially entails relational processing according to Bever, i.e., relating one kind of information to another. It is, he argues, 'an automatic conflict-resolving representation of reality' (p. 35) where 'we can reconcile apparently conflicting information by way of "inferences" about a possible world' (p. 33). Moving on from this definition of consciousness Bever suggests that:

> the processes underlying the empirical phenomena that distinguish the hemispheres are either unitary or relational. The effect of that difference is that the left hemisphere is more relational and hence more conscious (p. 34).

He concedes, however, that the right hemisphere is not entirely 'unconscious', but in an intact and integrated brain it is the left hemisphere which has control. Indeed, the left hemisphere may or may not be usefully characterized in terms of relational processing, but the problem with this view, as well as others, is that it reduces human consciousness to some form of cognitive processing. However, this depressing assumption is contrary to the clinical evidence which suggests that consciousness is not synonymous with cognition (Oakley, 1985).

Further support for the notion of dominance came from the fact that the great majority of individuals—between 88% and 95% according to most studies (Beaumont, 1974; Hardyck and Petrinovitch, 1977; Hicks and Kinsbourne, 1978)—are more efficient in the use of the right hand. A consequence of the contralateral organization of the nervous system is that each hemisphere controls the motor activity of the hand on the opposite side of the body and there are thought to be intimate relationships between the central control of speech and the central control of hand movement (Hécaen and Sauguet, 1971; Kimura and Dornford, 1974; Kertesz and Hooper, 1982). Both functions combine, therefore, to support the notion that for most of us the left hemisphere controls most mental activity.

The idea of dominance was challenged by Wigan (1844) and Jackson (1874). Jackson proposed that the left hemisphere might be considered the 'leading' hemisphere for propositional language, but that the right hemisphere was the leading hemisphere for visual processing. This notion of 'duality', where the two hemispheres had different but equal responsibilities, gained more recent support from Zangwill (1960), and particularly from a series of important papers that appeared in 1969 in the *Bulletin of the Los Angeles Neurological Societies* by Bogen (Bogen, 1969a,b; Bogen and Bogen, 1969). In the second of these papers Bogen develops the Jacksonian dual-brain notion of cerebral organization, where each hemisphere is seen as having different, but equal, cognitive capabilities, with the left operating in a propositional mode and the right in an 'appositional' mode. Research had concentrated on investigating left hemisphere capabilities and little was known about right hemisphere abilities, even as recently as 1969. Bogen considered that part of the value of the term appositional was that it represented little, but its fuller meaning would emerge as research into the role of the right hemisphere in the control of behaviour increased. Since 1969, and especially in recent years, there has grown what Lamendella (1977) called 'the cult of the right hemisphere' which is still amassing evidence from experimental and clinical studies to support the view that the right hemisphere has an equally important, if different, role in the control of mental activity.

In fact, as Bogen (1969b) points out, there is a long history of support for duality of function and the notion of left hemisphere dominance is a relatively recent idea.

> The likely explanation of the eclipse of the two-brain view was the emergence of the concept of cerebral dominance. The social disabilities of the dysphasic (especially in a society which emphasizes 'rational' thought) were so much more obvious than the defects of the right-brain-damaged person that dysphasia was accepted as a left hemisphere symptom, the right hemisphere was soon forgotten. And the increasing preoccupation of the neurologists with the peculiarities of the left hemisphere diverted them from a more comprehensive view (Bogen, 1969b, p. 153).

Gardner, Brownell, Wapner, and Michelow (1983) have also emphasized the tendency in the past for clinicians and researchers to focus their attention on the left hemisphere. Right-hemisphere-damaged patients did not show the marked impairments in cognition so obvious in many left-hemisphere-damaged individuals.

Thus although hardly ever tested in a thorough manner, the idea persisted that an individual's cognitive competence is clearly linked to the intactness of his left hemisphere, as did the corollary assumption that individuals with right hemisphere damage, their language apparently intact, are not seriously compromised in their ability to understand situations, solve problems, and make their way in the world (Gardner *et al.*, 1983, p. 171).

In 1974 Tueber was able to state that:

as nearly every contributor to the topic has stressed, the concept of unilateral dominance of the left by the right hemisphere in man has been abandoned and replaced by one of complementary specialization (Teuber, 1974, p. 71).

In contrast to the notion that the right hemisphere possesses little in the way of consciousness, Sperry (1984) holds a very different view. His interpretation of the research suggests that the right hemisphere is certainly conscious and he supports the concept of dual consciousness. He does not go along with those who propose that there exist two separate minds (Bogen, 1969a; Puccetti, 1973). Sperry (1984) has stated recently:

the conscious mind is normally single and unified, mediated by brain activity that spans and involves both hemispheres . . . the bilateral process can be viewed as an integrated dynamic entity that, functionally and causally, is qualitively different from, and more than, the mere sum of the left and right activities. In the normal state the two hemispheres function together as a very closely integrated whole, not as a double, divided, or bicameral system (p. 669).

A consequence of the increased interest in the right hemisphere is that we now have a more detailed appreciation of its role in mental activity. We will not attempt here to go over the functions of the right hemisphere in detail as so many good reviews are already available. (See, for instance, Hécaen and Albert, 1978; Perecman, 1983; Young, 1983.) We will be concerned in later chapters, however, to explore some functions which have particular relevance for the right hemisphere's contribution to communication.

It has been accepted for some time that the right hemisphere has special responsibility for visuospatial processing. To put it bluntly, despite constraints on interpretation due to methodological problems, there is 'no doubt that the case for right hemisphere superiority is not grounded in artifact' (Young and Ratcliff, 1983, p. 23). Using Marr's (1980) theory of human vision as a basis for interpretation, Young and Ratcliff recently concluded that the right hemisphere's visuospatial superiority emerges more for complex representational operations like form and object recognition and configuration, than for elementary lower level ('primal sketch') processing such as simple visual detection and localization. The evidence comes from studies on normal and brain damaged subjects. Damage to the right hemisphere often results in impairments in functions which appear to require intact visuospatial processing abilities. Patients may present with a range of disorders: these include constructional apraxias, where difficulties are experienced with the manipulation of objects in space to produce a three-dimensional structure or produce drawings of objects; prosopagnosia or facial agnosia, where patients experience problems in recognizing familiar faces; visual aspects of memory; tactile and visual recognition of complex geometric patterns; disorientation in space, which can be so severe that an individual is unable to find their way about their own home or comprehend depth and distance relationships; unilateral left-side neglect, which entails an apparent lack of awareness of the left side of the body and space, often in the absence of significant left visual-field impairments; sometimes related to left unilateral neglect is anosognosia—an indifference to or denial of impairment or illness. In the auditory modality, disorders of musical processing and other auditory agnosias for non-verbal sounds are observed. Many of these impairments are rarely observed following left hemisphere damage (Hecaen and Albert, 1978; Perecman, 1983; Young and Ratcliff, 1983).

Levy succinctly summarized the position in 1974 as follows:

> In considering the two sets of functions it appears that they may be logically incompatible. The right hemisphere synthesizes over space. The left hemisphere synthesizes over time. The right hemisphere notes visual similarities to the exclusion of conceptual similarities. The left hemisphere does the opposite. The right hemisphere perceives form, the left hemisphere detail. The right hemisphere codes sensory input in terms of images, the left hemisphere in terms of linguistic descriptions. The right hemisphere lacks a phonological analyser; the left hemisphere lacks a Gestalt analyser (Levy, 1974, p. 167).

Not only do the two hemispheres appear to be concerned in the processing of different functions, but many workers have attempted to characterize the hemispheres as *modal* processors, where two intrinsically different modes of information processing underlie the apparent functional specialization of each hemisphere. We shall see that much of the research in the area has been directed towards testing the predictions of these characterizations. There is a large literature which supports the complementary specialization concept and several attempts have been made to crystallize the essential form of the difference between the mental processing modes of the hemispheres. We have already referred to Bogen's (1969a) propositional–appositional dichotomy—based on Jackson's original propositional–non-propositional idea, and Bever's relational–unitary distinction. In addition to these. Semmes (1968) proposed that left hemisphere functions were more focally organized and structurally represented than functions processed predominantly by the right which were more diffusely organized and Nebes (1978) described the analytic left versus synthetic, holistic right hemisphere modes. Most of these dichotomous function notions have found a place in the analytic–holistic dichotomy (see Bradshaw and Nettleton, 1981, and accompanying comment for comprehensive review). At a more fundamental level, Bradshaw and Nettleton (1981) suggest that the research shows that the left hemisphere is specialized for temporal order, sequencing, and segmental processing:

Accordingly, the left hemisphere mediation of language is not seen to depend upon its symbolic or even largely phonological attributes, but upon the need for analytic, time-dependent, and sequential coding to occur, both at receptive, and more particularly, expressive levels (Bradshaw and Nettleton, 1981, p. 69). The fundamental cognitive skills of the right hemisphere, in contrast, are thought to be processing of the whole not the individual segments, the Gestalt not the sequence, the global features of mental experience, not the elements.

This book is concerned with the right hemisphere's role in human communication. Our concern will be with human communication in its wider sense, to encompass not only those formal linguistically describable components of language, but also such aspects of interaction as facial expression, paralinguistic features and extralinguistic features, including pragmatic aspects of communication. Neurolinguistic studies are carried out with a large range of subject groups using a variety of techniques, and in Chapter 2 we examine the problems of data interpretation that this produces. This relieves us of the necessity to refer constantly to these problems as discussion progresses. The reader with an appreciation of these difficulties in neuro-psychological research may skip Chapter 2. Chapter 3 concerns itself with the comprehension of strict linguistic aspects of language by the right hemisphere, Chapter 4 with non-linguistic and extralinguistic aspects of communication, and Chapter 5 with the expression and production of language. The motive for this division of labour is mainly practical and is not meant to support any particular system of classification or to emphasize boundaries between components of communication. Chapters 6 and 7 examine the contribution of the right hemisphere to the recovery of aphasia, and Chapter 8 its role in rehabilitation. Chapter 9 draws some general conclusions.

Marshall (1977) has proposed that 'the primary goal of neurolinguistic inquiry can be simply stated: the discipline seeks to understand the form of representation of language in the human brain' (p. 127). This book is concerned with the form of representation of language in one half of the brain—the right cerebral hemisphere.

Chapter Two

POPULATION AND METHODOLOGICAL VARIABLES IN RESEARCH INTO THE NEUROPSYCHOLOGY OF LANGUAGE

Our current understanding of relationships between language and brain comes from a wide range of populations examined using a variety of investigatory techniques. Most of what is known about hemispheric asymmetries in language processing comes from investigations with various clinical populations and often the data from different groups appear to be in conflict. This may be because the cerebral organization of the different groups varies and it may also be due to differences in the techniques of investigation used.

In fact, some studies have produced widely differing estimates of language lateralization between clinical and normal groups, attributed by Searleman (1977) to the fact that language *perception* is usually what is being estimated in normal subjects using the behavioural paradigms of dichotic listening and tachistoscopic hemi-field viewing, whereas language *production* is usually evaluated in clinical populations. While this may be a contributory factor, some studies which have compared perception between groups or production between groups have still found marked differences.

Studies on right hemisphere language have been conducted with a whole range of brain damaged as well as neurologically normal subjects. Each group has to be considered separately as it would appear questionable, *prima facie*, that the neural organization of language is the same in a right hemisphere which is separated from the left hemisphere and has a history of epilepsy (commissurotomy), a right hemisphere which stands in isolation (hemispherectomy or hemidecortication), a right hemisphere which has a damaged neighbour, and the right hemisphere of a normal brain. Different hypotheses concerning the neural organization of language are possible in each group.

Many of the most reliable and effective techniques used in assessing the language competence of the cerebral hemispheres involve not inconsiderable risk to the subject. Consequently, such tests are used only when the risk is considered unavoidable and necessary to guide surgery. For this reason, the tests are not used routinely with individuals free from neurological symptoms. From the point of view of understanding the right hemisphere's apparent role in language, it is therefore necessary to examine this role separately in the different populations.

The purpose of this chapter is to outline briefly the status and limitations of the principal neurophysiological and behavioural methods which have been used in neurolinguistic research, and to highlight the variability in the value of the data obtained from different populations. Some populations, techniques, and issues are considered in more detail than others, reflecting the relative importance of their contribution to the topic of this volume.

POPULATIONS

Unilateral brain damage

Observations on the presence or absence of impairment in language functions following unilateral brain damage (damage to one side of the brain) constitute the oldest and largest database in the study of the relationships between brain and language. However, the very mass of the literature poses problems of comparison between studies of variable quality.

Statements regarding the impairment of behaviour in unilaterally brain damaged patients are often made with little or no regard for the significant effects of such variables as aetiology, recovery patterns, and age of onset. Studies of aphasic patients with unilateral left hemisphere damage have been most commonly conducted on patients who have suffered a cerebrovascular accident (CVA) or traumatic injury to the brain. There are marked differences in size of lesion, age of onset, types of deficit, severity of aphasia and patterns of recovery in these two major groups. Constrast, for instance, the distinct approaches to the classification and theoretical explanation of aphasia by Schuell and co-workers and by Luria. Schuell's study (Schuell, Jenkins, and Jimenez-Pabon, 1964) was conducted primarily with CVA patients and Luria's (1970) with patients who had sustained missile wounds to the brain. There are major differences in aphasia due to CVA and trauma which do not allow the easy pooling of data from the two groups. Patients who have sustained traumatic injury to the brain are generally much younger than CVA patients as a group; war injuries occur predominantly in young males, and closed head injuries following road traffic accidents also occur mainly in children, adolescents, and young adults (Levin, 1981); while CVAs occur mainly in individuals between 40 and 70 years (Davis and Holland, 1981).

Recovery patterns and levels of recovery differ between these two main groups, with post-traumatic patients generally making a better recovery than post-CVA patients. Global aphasia secondary to CVA is usually irreversible (Schuell et al. 1964), although there are exceptions; global aphasia due to trauma can recover to a mild anomic aphasia (Kertesz, 1979; Levin, 1981). The area of brain destroyed by a penetrating missile wound is generally more focally concentrated than the lesion caused by a CVA.

Even within these two main groups there are differences in aetiology and type of brain damage. 'CVA' itself is a term used to encompass a range of possible disorders of cerebrovascular origin, including cerebral thrombosis, embolism, haemorrhage, vascular malformations, and various others, all with different clinical signs and effects upon behaviour. Traumatic damage to the brain can be caused either by relatively focal penetrating open head injuries (where there is actual penetration causing laceration to brain tissue), or closed head injuries where a significant cause of damage is rotational acceleration of the skull (producing shearing and stretching of tissue and damage caused by the brain being thrust against the skull). In addition the nature of aphasic impairment due to closed head injury is different to aphasia secondary to CVA; in closed head injury anomia and Wernicke's aphasia predominate with non-fluent agrammatic Broca's aphasia being relatively rare (Levin, 1981).

In investigations of unilaterally left-hemisphere-damaged individuals, subjects are often grouped according to aphasia type on the basis of performance on an aphasia battery. There are marked differences in age and rates and patterns of recovery in various clinical types of aphasia. Broca's aphasic patients as a group have been found to be significantly younger than Wernicke's patients (discussed more fully later in this chapter); a factor which should confound attempts to age-match subjects in separate experimental groups. The rate of recovery made by Broca's patients is reported to be highest (Kertesz and McCabe, 1977; Kertesz, 1979) although anomic and conduction patients present initially with less severe impairments and are more likely to make complete recoveries. Initially, globally impaired patients, with some exceptions, make poor recoveries (Schuell et al. 1964) and the pattern of recovery for Wernicke's patients is the most variable (Kertesz, 1979). A further confounding factor in aphasia research, often overlooked in grouping patients into subtypes, is the degree to which patients can evolve from one clinical aphasia type to another with time and recovery. In his study of 93 aphasic patients, Kertesz (1979) found that of 22 global patients 2 evolved into Broca's and 3 into either transcortical motor, conduction or anomic; of 17 patients initially classified as Broca's 3 evolved into anomic and 1 into transcortical motor; of 8 patients originally diagnosed as conduction, 5 made complete recoveries and 2 ended up as anomic; of 13 Wernicke's patients, 4 became anomic and 2 became either global or transcortical sensory. The rest of the series were made up of transcortical motor, sensory, and anomic patients ($N = 33$), 19 of which made either complete recoveries or evolved into anomic patients. Of 90 patients, 79 'evolved' from initial classification.

It seems probable that the difficulties of comparison and failures of replication in aphasia research, as well as the lack of agreement regarding the efficacy of treatment, owe much to our ignorance concerning the interactions of the confounding variables outlined above. This heterogeneity of the aphasic population needs to be borne in mind when comparing data from different studies.

Commissurotomy

Given the enormous impact that the pioneering 'split-brain' work of Sperry, Bogen, Gazzaniga, and others (Sperry, 1961, 1964; Gazzaniga, Bogen, and Sperry, 1962; Sperry, Gazzaniga, and Bogen, 1969) has had on views of brain–behaviour relationships, hemispheric asymmetry and the mind–body problem, it is interesting to note that the first examinations of patients who had undergone sectioning of the corpus callosum in the early 1940s revealed no interference with the normal functioning of language (Searleman, 1977; Walsh, 1978). In fact, until the mid-1960s it was generally believed that the right hemisphere was not involved in language at all (Gazzaniga, 1977). This provided some support to Lashley's (1929) notorious, and not entirely facetious remark, that the sole function of the corpus callosum was to hold the two hemispheres together. There was even the waggish suggestion that its function was to allow seizures to spread from one hemisphere to the other. However, since the early days more sophisticated testing methods have been developed and the split-brain work has produced important information concerning the verbal abilities and limitations of the right hemisphere. In fact, it is mostly due to this work that there has been a re-emergence of the duality hypothesis.

Despite, or maybe because of, the impact of the commissurotomy findings, split-brain research has come in for some fierce criticism in more recent years. It should be recalled that the operation has been carried out on very few individuals and the entire but extensive commissurotomy literature is based on a mere handful of individual cases (Gazzaniga, 1983). The limitations of single-case study research, discussed on page 12 in this chapter, therefore apply. The major criticism of the research is that the findings must at least be viewed with considerable reservation or even completely discounted, on the grounds that the data give a false impression of the hemispheric capabilities of the normal brain.

The major problem is that the commissurotomy operation is usually only undertaken in cases where the patient has suffered severe epilepsy for many years (usually since childhood), due to a large lesion. The surgery is carried out in an attempt to prevent the spread of the epileptic seizure from one hemisphere to the other. The patients had therefore experienced significant brain damage in early life which in all probability had caused major functional reorganization.

The operation itself involves cutting the corpus callosum which joins the two hemispheres, and sometimes other commissural connections. Subcortical connections between the two hemispheres are left intact. The surgery entails a fairly brutal insult to the brain, as Millar and Whitaker (1983) have recently emphasized:

> One hemisphere (usually the non-dominant) is pulled aside to expose the corpus callosum; a large number of arteries and veins which run between the two

hemispheres are coagulated; and the corpus callosum (and occasionally one or more interhemispheric commissures) is divided almost totally. The operation itself causes some brain damage, inevitably. Pulling aside one hemisphere (retraction) bruises the hemisphere along the mesial (inside, or middle) surface; coagulating the bridging arteries and veins causes the death of tissue supplies by those arteries and veins (pp. 102–103).

In addition to the damage caused by the operation itself, there is a high probability that the patient has a history of early brain damage to one hemisphere or the other which may have caused substantial functional reorganization; the nature of which will depend upon the hemispheric site of the epileptic lesion. Millar and Whitaker (1983, p. 104) summarize succinctly the hypothetical effects of early damage to one or other hemisphere:

> if the epileptic lesion is in the right hemisphere, it . . . obviously cannot subserve language functions normally. Therefore, any evaluation of language functions in the right hemisphere will fall short of what an unimpaired right hemisphere could do. If . . . [the] epileptic lesion is in the left hemisphere however . . . some language functions will probably have transferred over to the right hemisphere. Therefore, any evaluation of language functions in the right hemisphere will exaggerate, or overestimate, what the normal right hemisphere does. The obvious conclusion is that one cannot assess right hemisphere language functions in the split-brain patient.

Despite such fierce criticisms the split-brain research has produced interesting, if controversial findings. Clearly there are limitations to the contribution that the research can make to our understanding of language functions in the normal brain. (See the recent exchange between Gazzaniga, 1983; Levy, 1983; and Zaidel, 1983.) However, the findings do make a contribution to our understanding of the effects of early left hemisphere brain damage on the reorganizational capabilities of the brain, especially with reference to the potential linguistic competence of the right hemisphere following left hemisphere damage.

Hemispherectomy and hemidecortication

Hemispherectomy describes the complete surgical removal of a cerebral hemisphere, whereas the term hemidecortication implies the removal of the lobes of the neocortex while leaving intact subcortical nuclear masses such as the thalamus and components of the basal ganglia. However, the term hemispherectomy is still used quite widely to describe both surgical procedures, although it should perhaps be reserved to indicate complete removal of cortical and subcortical tissue. The distinction becomes especially important where discussion of the role of the remaining isolated hemisphere in specific cognitive functions is concerned.

These radical procedures are usually performed on either adults suffering from large life-threatening neoplastic tumours or on children to reduce the effects of infantile hemiplegia. The evidence concerning lateralization of language functions in the brain derived from studies on patients who have undergone this major surgery therefore addresses two separate but related questions: the lateralization of language functions in the developing brain and the lateralization of language functions in the mature adult brain. The contribution of the infantile hemispherectomy and hemidecortication studies towards understanding the relationship between brain ontogeny and lateralization of language functions is discussed later. It is concluded below that the quality of most of the evidence is such that firm results cannot be drawn. What reliable evidence there is, however, does not support the equipotentiality hypothesis. From the point of view of improving our understanding of the lateralization of language functions in the mature brain, clearly both the quality and the nature of the evidence from childhood studies is deficient. Not only do the adult and childhood groups differ in age of surgery, and age of onset of disease, but also in background neurological aetiology. The contribution to our knowledge of studies with mature subjects is considered in detail in Chapters 3 and 4.

The hemispherectomy and hemidecortication evidence suffers from similar deficiencies as the commissurotomy evidence: the individuals being examined have both suffered severe, if different, neurological disorders, and both groups undergo radical surgical invasion of the brain. There is a difference, however, in the quality of the studies: the detail and care taken in examining and reporting on language functions in many of the hemispherectomy and hemidecortication patients is disappointing.

Individual differences

A major research method in neuropsychology, from Broca's original studies right up to the commissurotomy, hemispherectomy, and hemidecortication studies of recent times, is the single-case study. In fact, it is not an exaggeration to say that much of our current understanding of brain–behaviour relationships comes from detailed investigation of a series of individual cases.

Data obtained thus, clearly have limitations. As Millar and Whitaker (1983) observe:

> from the case history one answers the question 'Is it possible for such-and-such to occur?' From the case history one does *not* answer the question 'Does everyone exhibit such-and-such?'

Individual differences must be borne in mind when interpreting data, especially when comparing data between studies and particularly data from single cases or a handful of single cases. Such individual differences as sex, handedness, familial sinistrality, age, actual brain morphology, early experience and literacy (see Segalowitz and Bryden, 1983, for a recent comprehensive review), as well, no doubt, as others not yet implicated, are not always controlled for in experimental studies and often their possible influence is overlooked in interpretation of data from single cases. Bogen (Bogen, De Zure, Houten, and Marsh, 1972; Bogen and Bogen, 1983) has proposed the notion of 'hemisphericity' to account for many of the individual differences apparent in the cerebral organization of functions in different individuals. On this hypothesis a function may be more or less lateralized and more or less focally organized within a hemisphere in an individual brain, depending on such factors as past environmental experience, individual cognitive styles, individual cognitive strategies, individual levels of skill and appreciation, and even time of day and time of life. This may be appreciated by considering the results of studies which have examined dichotic ear advantages for various aspects of music in skilled musicians and non-musicians. Findings suggest that there are marked differences in the cognitive organization and lateralization of music depending on levels of skill and appreciation between individuals. Such studies are discussed more fully in Chapter 5. There are also indications that the organization and lateralization of language vary individually depending on similar factors and these are discussed below. Beaumont, Young, and McManus (1984) have recently suggested that the hemisphericity theory can be abandoned as there is little or no good scientific support for the idea.

The problem of individual differences is a major one in neuropsychology, and an adequate theory is still a long way off. As Marshall (1973) has stated it, such a theory would need to:

> specify how different subjects set up different computational modes (which may well be associated with relatively circumscribed locales) in different orders and with different weightings. The *a priori* likelihood that all subjects approach clinical tests in the same way is not very great; this in turn is presumably not unrelated to the notorious lack of repeatability that characterizes many branches of the psychology of higher cognitive functions (p. 467).

The most widely investigated and often implicated individual differences are those of sex, age, and handedness.

Sex

The mass of evidence seems to support the notion that there are significant differences in hemispheric organization of language between males and females. Results of unilateral brain damage studies (McGlone, 1977, 1978; see McGlone, 1980, for review) as well as studies with normal subjects (see Bryden, 1979, for review) support the view that language is more bilaterally represented in females than in males.

McGlone (1978, 1980) tested unilaterally brain damaged male and female patients on the WAIS. She found a significant reduction in Verbal IQ but not Performance IQ in left-hemisphere-damaged male subjects but not in females, and a significant deficit in Performance IQ in right-hemisphere-damaged males, but not females. The average Verbal IQ for left-hemisphere-damaged male subjects was 86.5 and for left-hemisphere-damaged females 100.6. In right-hemisphere-damaged subjects, the average Verbal IQ was 100.5 for males and 98.4 for females.

A number of dichotic studies with normal subjects have found that females are more likely to produce a left ear advantage (LEA) than a right ear advantage (REA) in comparison with male subjects (Bryden, 1966; Briggs and Nebes, 1976; Lake and Bryden, 1976), although several studies have failed to demonstrate these clear sex differences (see Bryden, 1979, for full review). Similarly, a number of tachistoscopic studies have reported sex differences, generally in the direction of increased right visual-field (RVF) advantage in males when compared to females, on a variety of tasks (Hannay and Malone, 1976; Segalowitz and Stewart, 1979), although again there are exceptions to this general finding (Bryden, 1979). The underlying character of the observed sex differences on experimental tasks following brain damage may not necessarily be concerned with laterality *per se*, however. Segalowitz and Bryden (1983) suggest that the sex differences reported in dichotic studies, for instance, may depend on the degree of control exercised over the subjects' freedom in choosing the way in which they deploy their attention. Sex differences observed on laterality tasks may indicate strategic differences, rather than language lateralization differences between the sexes. They conclude:

> If men and women adopt different ways of approaching a particular task, we cannot be sure whether to attribute sex differences in laterality to differences in the cerebral representation of language processes or to differences in the strategy employed. For this reason it is particularly important to understand the experimental procedure being employed and to attempt to control individual differences in strategy (Segalowitz and Bryden, 1983, p. 363).

Age

The major concern with the effects of age on experimental and clinical data is the degree to which hemispheric involvement in the processing of particular functions may vary with time of life. There are problems with the data derived from studies of children, especially as controversy rages over whether it is the case that language is lateralized to the left hemisphere at birth, or whether the newborn baby starts with a hemispheric bilateral potential for language which gradually lateralizes to the left with development.

Lenneberg (1967) is most associated with the latter of these positions and based his arguments on the observation by Basser (1962) that acquired aphasia in children is less severe and more often transitory than in adults, and damage to either hemisphere in children between 2 and 5 years will cause aphasia. This latter claim was also adopted and extended by Krashen (1972). The argument goes that aphasia is less severe because only some aspects of language are affected by a unilateral lesion, other aspects being represented in the other hemisphere; the aphasia is transitory because the undamaged hemisphere soon compensates for the damaged one. Aphasia will result from damage to either hemisphere because language is represented in both. Lenneberg suggested that these observations support the cerebral plasticity hypothesis: the view that the cerebral hemispheres are equipotential for language in children, and damage to the left hemisphere would result in substantial compensation by the right hemisphere.

The hypothesis that there exists bilateral representation for language in children has been criticized on a number of counts by Kinsbourne and Hiscock (1977) and the traditional plasticity hypothesis, based to a large extent on early childhood hemispherectomy and hemidecortication studies, is not supported by more recent interpretations of this data (Dennis and Whitaker, 1976; Satz and Bullard-Bates, 1981; St James-Roberts, 1979, 1981). These recent reinterpretations draw quite the contrary conclusion in fact: infantile left hemispherectomy does indeed cause a retardation in language development, and the right hemisphere is not capable of developing the full linguistic capabilities of the left hemisphere.

St James-Roberts (1981) resubmitted the great mass of childhood hemispherectomy studies to re-examination. His conclusions suggest that Basser's (1962) influential study, upon which Lenneberg (1967) based much of his argument, was deficient in the quality of its reporting, relying to a large degree on anecdotal evidence. The childhood hemispherectomy literature, St James-Roberts suggests, prevents valid comparisons being made between studies due to such additional shortcomings as:

> failure to control test procedures, the status of the residual nervous system, diaschisis variables, recovery periods and experimental variables, all of which contribute to brain damage recovery measures (p. 47).

Where such variables are taken into account and patients are compared:

> neither age at brain damage nor hemisphere damaged predicts verbal or performance IQs consistently, and although some age-group effects have been found for IQ differences scores in right hemispherectomies, these are neither compelling nor consistent with the predictions of the plasticity hypothesis (pp. 47–48).

In fact, individual differences in aetiology and test variables seem to influence recovery scores more than the variables of age or hemisphere damaged.

Another recent critical review of the childhood aphasia literature (Satz and Bullard-Bates, 1981) arrived at the following conclusions:

1. The risk of aphasia or language impairment is approximately the same in right-handed children and adults if the left hemisphere is damaged.
2. The risk of aphasia or language impairment is substantially greater following left versus right-sided brain injury regardless of age—at least after infancy.
3. The risk of aphasia after right hemisphere injury (crossed aphasia) is rare in both right-handed adults and children, particularly after ages 3–5 years and perhaps earlier.
4. The aphasia pattern, while predominantly non-fluent in a majority of children, is by no means invariant. As with adults, other aphasic patterns can coexist or appear independently, including disorders of auditory comprehension, writing, reading, and naming. . . .

5. Spontaneous recovery, while dramatic in a majority of children, is by no means invariant. A majority of studies disclosed a number of unremitting cases (25–50%) after 1 year post-onset. Furthermore, even in cases of recovery from aphasia, serious cognitive and academic sequelae were found (p. 421).

The quality of much of the childhood aphasia evidence is questionable but those conclusions that can be drawn seriously undermine the foundations of the childhood plasticity hypothesis. As Dennis and Whitaker (1976) conclude:

Hemispheric equipotentiality does appear to make an untenable supposition about the brain because it neither explains nor predicts at least two facts about language—that the two perinatal hemispheres are not equally at risk for language delay or disorder and that they are not equivalent substrates for language acquisition (p. 103).

Regard for age as a factor which should be considered when interpreting data from adult populations is underscored by the observation that aphasia type following unilateral left hemisphere damage due to CVA is to some extent influenced by the age of onset. Obler, Albert, Goodglass, and Benson (1978) examined the relationships between age and onset of aphasia in 167 CVA patients. They found that, while global conduction and anomic patients clustered around the median age of 55.8 years, Wernicke's patients were significantly older (median age 63 years) and Broca's patients significantly younger (median age 51 years) than the group median. Secondly, the incidence of Wernicke's aphasia appears to rise with increasing age, while the incidence of other aphasia types increases to a peak between 52 and 57 years, and then decreases with increasing age. De Renzi, Faglioni, and Ferrari (1980) examined the same relationships between age and aphasia type in 200 patients (177 CVA, 23 tumour). Patients were grouped into global, Broca's (including transcortical motor), and Wernicke's (including transcortical sensory) and the study also found Broca's patients (mean age 56.8 years) to be significantly younger than Wernicke's patients (mean age 62.6 years). Brown and Jaffe (Brown and Jaffe, 1975; Brown, 1976, 1979) have proposed a 'continuing lateralization' hypothesis where hemispheric specialization is seen to develop through life from infancy to late adulthood, and it is this which accounts for the age–aphasia type interactions which have been observed. On this hypothesis, aphasia type can be predicted by an interaction between degree of left hemisphere specialization and site of lesion. It is proposed that a different neural substrate for language exists in the brain at different ages. However, Obler et al. (1978) make the point that other explanations are possible. Posterior lesions may increase with age because the posterior cerebrovascular system itself is more prone to compromise in later life; changes in cognition and cognitive style related to ageing may intereact to produce a Wernicke's type of aphasia irrespective of the precise site of lesion within the left hemisphere language areas. It may also be of significance that the language problems of individuals suffering from cortical forms of dementia due to general atrophy of the brain mirror closely the behavioural pattern of Wernicke's aphasia due to a left posterior temporal lesion. However, Kertesz and Sheppard (1981) suggest that surveys of chronic patients where time since onset was not controlled could bias results in favour of differences being found. Their own study was on 192 patients who were examined within 48 days post-onset and for the majority of whom brain and/or CT scan verification of site of lesion was available. This study found no significant differences between age and aphasia type.

Other factors relating to age and aphasia, which are often uncontrolled for in aphasia research, have recently been reviewed by Davis and Holland (1981). While the peak incidence for CVA is between 40 and 70 years, that of the most common brain tumour in adults is between 45 and 55 years. Traumatic head injuries caused by road traffic accidents can, of course, occur at any age (although there is a higher incidence in young adulthood), with war injuries occurring predominantly in young men. Clearly, any use of aphasic data to examine questions concerning the cerebral organization of language must take these factors into account. As Davis and Holland (1981, p. 210) conclude:

> the interaction of etiology and age complicate any attempt to establish general descriptions of aphasia because different etiologies produce different recovery patterns.

Handedness
Despite extensive study, difficulties still exist concerning the precise specification of the relationships between handedness and hemispheric representation for language. What is known is that handedness is a major variable related to hemispheric organization of language, and, as indicated earlier (Chapter 1), there are thought to be intimate relationships between the cerebral control of praxis and language (Hécaen and Sauguet, 1971; Kimura and Archibald, 1974; Kertesz and Hooper, 1982; Mateer, 1983).

The overwhelming majority of right-handed individuals, making up between 88% and 96% of the population according to most studies (Beaumont, 1974; Hardyck and Petrinovitch, 1977; Rasmussen and Milner, 1977; Hicks and Kinsbourne, 1978; Segalowitz and Bryden, 1983) have left hemisphere specialization for language (Milner, Branch, and Rasmussen, 1966; Rasmussen and Milner, 1977), as well as most left-handers. A small proportion of right-handers (4% according to Rasmussen and Milner, 1977) have right hemisphere specialization for language (for speech production at least) as demonstrated by the rare incidence of crossed aphasia (aphasia in a right-handed individual following a unilateral right hemisphere lesion). This leaves a percentage of left-handers who appear to have right hemisphere specialization or bilateral representation for language. Satz's (1980) review of the handedness and aphasia literature concluded that bilateral representation in left-handers may be as high as 40%; an incidence much higher than indicated by other studies. Using the sodium amytal technique, Rasmussen and Milner (1977) found that 96% of right-handers had left hemisphere specialization for speech (4% being right-hemisphere specialized) while 15% of left-handers have right hemisphere specialization and 15% have bilateral representation. These figures compare well with Segalowitz and Bryden's (1983) recent estimate based on a more selective review of the clinical literature. The presence of familial sinistrality has been implicated as a factor which may help explain why some left-handers have left hemisphere representation while others have right hemisphere representation for language (Hácaen and Sauguet, 1971; Hardyck and Petrinovitch, 1977), although the evidence is inconclusive.

Hardyck and Petrinovitch (1977) concluded from their analysis of the handedness literature that individuals who are clearly right-handed with no family history of left-handedness are the most strongly left-hemisphere lateralized and that most left-handers with no family history of left-handedness are also left-hemisphere specialized for language. However, left-handers who have a positive family history of sinistrality are the most likely to have bilateral representation for language. It is this latter group who recover much more quickly and show fewer lasting effects of brain damage.

Individual and familial handedness are important factors to be taken into consideration in discussions of hemispheric processing of language. A number of studies have shown that such factors can have a significant influence on recovery from aphasia (Subirana, 1958; Gloning, Gloning, Haube, and Quatember, 1969; Hécaen and Sauguet, 1971; Hardyck and Petrinovitch, 1977; Hicks and Kinsbourne, 1978) as well as significantly affecting the performance of normal subjects on dichotic listening (Satz, Achenbach, Pattishall, and Fennell, 1965; Curry, 1967; Searleman, 1980) and tachistoscopic viewing tasks (Bryden, 1965; 1973; Bradshaw and Taylor, 1979; Schmuller and Goodman, 1979). There are indications that handedness changes with age. Bingley's (1958) review estimated that the incidence of left-handedness in normal children entering school was approximately 8% decreasing to 5% to 6% in normal adults. Sand and Taylor's (1973) study suggested significantly increased mixed-handedness and a decreasing incidence of left-handedness with increasing age. Such studies seem to indicate, therefore, that there is a gradual shift from left- to right-handedness with increasing age. Borod and Goodglass (1980) have made the point, however, that such trends may have more to do with changing cultural patterns in the tolerance of left-handedness. The importance of the complicating factor of handedness, which plagues much neuropsychological research, has been emphasized by Hardyck and Petrinovitch (1977; p. 398) as follows:

> Handedness is not a simple phenomenon that is easily determined phenomenologically or by self-report. The development of preferred handedness

can be markedly affected by such factors as family and cultural preferences, educational practices, the prevalence of certain types of devices more suitable for one hand than the other, genetic factors, and specific brain damage, to mention only the immediately obvious items.

NEUROPHYSIOLOGICAL METHODS

The Sodium Amytal Method

The sodium amytal or Wada (1949) method is generally considered to be the most reliable method yet available for determining lateralization of function in the brain. The use of this technique is primarily associated with Milner and her associates at the Montreal Neurological Institute (Milner, Branch, and Rasmussen, 1968; Milner, 1974) where several hundred cases have been tested. It involves the injection of, usually, 200 mg of 10% sodium amytal, a fast acting barbiturate, into first the carotid artery on one side and then the carotid artery on the other side on two separate occasions. The sodium amytal acts to anaesthetize most of the hemisphere ipsilateral to the side of the injection for between 5 and 10 minutes and produces the expected contralateral hemiplegia, hemisensory loss, and hemianopia. If the hemisphere specialized for speech is anaesthetized the patient is usually mute for about 2 minutes following which he or she begins to make typical aphasic errors on naming objects with verbal perseverations, paraphasias, and jargon. Errors occur also in counting backwards or in recitation of the days of the week backwards, as well as occasional mistakes on simple reading tasks.

Due to the possible dangers inherent in the method it is usually reserved for investigations of patients being prepared for neurosurgery, in order to help establish the hemisphere specialized for language processing and other functions. Consequently, most of the data concerning lateralization of functions obtained with the sodium amytal technique is from subjects who are not neurologically 'normal', and may consequently have undergone a certain amount of cerebral and cognitive reorganization. A further problem is that the injected sodium amytal does not only affect the ipsilateral hemisphere, but can pass to the contralateral hemisphere and the resulting behavioural impairment observed on testing may not be 100% reliably caused by anaesthetization of the ipsilateral hemisphere. None the less, despite these drawbacks, the technique is considered to be the most reliable one available at the moment for examining lateralization of functions in the brain.

Computerized tomography

The introduction of computerized tomography (CT) scanning has had a significant effect upon our ability to correlate the site and extent of brain lesions with functional deficits, especially in the area of aphasia. The technique is anatomically based; it provides information on structural anatomical changes in tissue. In the typical examination, 8 to 10 consecutive cross-sectional X-ray 'slices' (10 mm thick), are taken and damaged brain tissue shows up as being darker than intact tissue. In this way, the site and extent of a lesion can be observed through most dimensions (Naeser, 1983). The quantification of lesion size can be determined by computer count of the actual number of 'pixels' (usually 1 mm × 1 mm picture elements) contained within a lesion or by calculating the relative percentage of hemisphere tissue damage (the left hemisphere can be compared to the right hemisphere). Naeser (1983, p. 67), in her comprehensive review, states that:

> the number of pixels in a lesion can be obtained in less than 1 minute on most CT scanners available today (without the Automatic Framing Program—AFP). The investigator merely calls up the 'irregular regions of interest' or 'map' function program at the CRT viewer screen, and traces over the lesion with the joy-stick controlled marker. The pixels are automatically counted and the total instantly appears on the CRT.

Further detailed explanations of the CT scan technique can be found in Naeser and Hayward (1978), Naeser, Hayward, Laughlin, and Zatz (1981), and Naeser (1983).

The technique has contributed much to our understanding of brain damage–behaviour correlates. With regard to cortical aphasias, at least, highly significant correlations are observed between lesion size and severity of aphasia. Such high correlations are not observed with subcortical aphasias, atypical aphasias, multiple lesion cases, and bilateral lesions (Naeser, 1983). The quality of the information derived from CT scan studies depends upon such factors as quality of case history information, clinical description of behavioural deficits, and time since onset of lesion. A major drawback of the technique is that it is able to provide quantification of site and extent of lesion only at the time of actual evaluation. Other techniques, however, can provide *in vivo* information.

Positron emission tomography

Positron emission tomography (PET) and positron emission-computed tomography (PECT) are variants of a relatively new and potentially powerful technique (Benson, Metter, Kuhl, and Phelps, 1983). This is a 'non-invasive' scanning technique which produces a cross-sectional image of radioactivity in the brain. The technique can potentially measure metabolism, bloodflow, and other activities in brain tissue depending on the radioactive indicator which is intravenously injected. It therefore provides more than structural anatomical information. It is claimed that PET scanning is potentially more powerful than CT scanning in so far as it is able to show abnormalities actually within tissue, which, according to CT scanning, is structurally intact (Benson *et al.*, 1983). A further important advantage over the CT scan is that, like regional cerebral bloodflow (rCBF) described in a later section, it is able to provide information *in vivo*. A further potential advantage, however, is that it also provides information on subcortical tissue.

Early indications are that PET scanning can show alterations in metabolic activity following visual (Phelps, Kuhl, and Mazziotta, 1980) or auditory (Mazziotta, Phelps, Carson, and Kuhl, 1982) stimulation. The latter study, for instance, showed increased metabolic activity in the left temporal lobe during verbal, and the right temporal lobe during melodic, stimulation. Metter, Wasterlain, Kuhl, Hanson, and Phelps (1981) compared PECT evaluation of metabolic rate for glucose with CT anatomical information in five aphasic patients and found that PECT evaluation of metabolism showed areas of damage not detected by the CT anatomical data. Suppression of metabolism in undamaged brain tissue was also found which suggests that:

> Infarcted tissue may have widespread effects on structurally intact tissue . . . in areas synaptically connected to the damaged area. These metabolic changes may have functional importance (Metter *et al.*, 1981, pp. 181–182).

The technique holds promise for examining metabolic activity in deep-brain structures during controlled experimental situations, which should increase our understanding of the role of subcortical structures in behaviour.

Electroencephalography

Electroencephalography (EEG) is a technique which is fraught with problems, although those involved in its development suggest enthusiastically that it is *potentially* a powerful investigatory technique. Beaumont (1983; p. 225) suggests, for instance, that with the application of EEG,

> for the first time it is possible to observe in real time, that is, as they happen, cognitive processes and the physiological events which are believed to be associated with them. Thus for the first time we have a technique which may make it possible to construct a bridge between mental and physiological events. If so, then we have a solution to the problem which has dogged so much of neuropsychology, that of directly investigating mind–body relationships.

However, Beaumont goes on to warn that although the technique is promising for the future, major problems exist which make it as yet unreliable:

> it has to be said that there are a number of difficult technical problems to be solved with these methods of investigation, and there is not as yet any case in which a cognitive process has been shown to be associated unequivocally with a specific brain event (p. 225).

The interested reader is referred to Beaumont (1982, 1983) and Cooper, Ossleton, and Shaw (1980) for detailed discussion on the application of EEG. What follows is drawn from Beaumont's (1983) excellent introduction to the technique.

The two principal forms of EEG used in neuropsychological experiments are ongoing and evoked potential. Ongoing EEG entails the recording of the potential differences between pairs of silver cup electrodes place on the scalp with a third electrode placed elsewhere on the head acting as an earth. A pair of electrodes constitutes a single channel and typically a number of pairs of electrodes are positioned over the areas of brain to be investigated. The signals are amplified and computer processed and may be printed on a chart recorder.

The problems of interpreting the EEG signals associated with brain activity include interference from tissue other than brain tissue surrounding the electrodes, decisions regarding the contribution of a pair of electrodes to a change in potential difference, and the major problem of underlying asymmetrics of the brain. Regarding this latter difficulty Beaumont (1983; p. 229) states:

> we know that the brain is asymmetrical, particularly in certain regions, and there is a strong suspicion that these asymmetries have functional significance, but electrodes are applied to symmetrical points on the scalp. If we detect asymmetries in the EEG at homolateral points, do these represent lateral asymmetries in the activity of homolateral regions or merely indicate that we are recording from anatomically homolateral points on the brain? This is an extremely worrying problem, which, until we can determine individual differences in anatomical asymmetries, is insoluble.

The problems of EEG do not end here. There is also, for instance, ignorance concerning the actual relationship of the various wave types (Delta, Theta, Alpha, Beta 1, Beta 2) to actual mental events.

The measurement of evoked potentials (EPs) or averaged evoked potentials (AEPs) constitutes the other major variant of EEG. With this technique a simple sensory stimulus is presented a large number of times (up to 512). Data are collected by computer and averaged and analysed. The same problems plague EP as ongoing EEG research, with the major one being ignorance about what the data actually mean.

Both techniques are widely represented in the neuropsychological literature, but Beaumont warns that:

> close inspection of the reported results also reveals little unanimity about the precise effects to be observed, and there is little replication of experimental findings ... our ignorance about what to look for in either EEG or EP components means that it is almost impossible to construct sound experimental tests of precise neuropsychological hypotheses (p. 243).

In conclusion, this complex technique is not at a stage of development where it can answer questions concerning the contribution of a hemisphere in structured experimental sessions involving even relatively simple cognitive stimuli.

Regional Cerebral Bloodflow

The regional cerebral bloodflow (rCBF) technique is based on the observation that bloodflow through brain tissue varies as a function of metabolism and the actual functional activity of brain tissue. The bloodstream carries oxygen to brain tissue and an increased demand by tissue for oxygen causes an increase in bloodflow. The method detects changes in local nerve-cell activity via these changes in bloodflow caused by increased metabolic rate (Lassen, Ingvar, and Skinhoj, 1978).

A computer is programmed so that different degrees of departure from a resting state in bloodflow are displayed over a template of the cortex. Different coloured pixels (picture elements) a square centimetre in size represent different levels of bloodflow and hence metabolic rate and functional activity. A radioactive isotope of the inert gas *xenon* is either injected into one of the main arteries to the brain, or inhaled by the patient; and the course of the isotope through the brain is followed (for about 1 minute) by a gamma-ray camera having 254 detectors, each of which scans an area of about 1 square centimetre. This information is processed by computer and the processed detail of each detector is represented on a monitor screen as a 1 centimetre coloured square. Different colours represent different levels of bloodflow related to metabolic rate, and by inference functional activity. It is claimed that the method is relatively safe and provides a great deal of useful information concerning the behaviour of bloodflow on the superficial surface of the cortex during various activities. The technique is used, like others, for neurological examination of patients with suspected CVA, tumours or epilepsy, but despite this, it is claimed that some 80 normal brains have been studied. These patients, it is stated, were suffering transient neurological symptoms which were subsequently found to be unrelated to any brain abnormality (Lassen *et al.*, 1978). The major disadvantage of the technique is that it provides information only on superficial cortical activity and not deep-brain activity and the 1 minute or so available for testing does not allow detailed investigation of activity during complex cognitive tasks.

Electrical stimulation

The use of electrical stimulation of exposed areas of the brain in neuropsychology owes a great deal to the work of Penfield and co-workers (Penfield and Jasper, 1954; Penfield and Perot, 1963; Penfield and Roberts, 1959) at the Montreal Neurological Institute. The technique is employed during radical neurosurgery, and has proved valuable in determining which areas of brain in an individual are important for various functions, and should consequently be spared. The main patient groups are those undergoing stereotaxic thalamotomies for the relief of dyskinesia or intractable pain (Ojemann, 1983; Mateer and Ojemann, 1983) and surgical resection of medically untreatable epileptic foci predominantly in the anterior temporal lobe (Mateer, 1983).

The technique itself involves the application of an alternating electric current (produced by a constant-current stimulator) via either monopolar or bipolar silver-ball electrodes (Ojemann, 1983). Stimulation durations can be varied up to 15 seconds and can generate both inhibitory and excitatory effects:

> conduction in some fibres may be blocked, while nearby cell bodies may be excited. Elsewhere, fibres may be excited while activity in cell bodies may be inhibited by direct depolarization or propagated inhibitory effects from activated cell bodies elsewhere (inhibitory surround). Excitatory effects may be propagated antidromically or orthodromically, evoking either excitation or inhibition at a distance. Thus, direct physiologic prediction of the effects of stimulation—whether excitatory or inhibitory or both, and where they will occur—is not realistic (Ojemann, 1983, p. 190).

A special feature of the technique is that it appears to have very discrete and local effects; this constitutes a major advantage over all other methods of investigation. Furthermore,

> stimulation of one cortical site will alter a language function such as naming on every trial, while stimulation at the same current at a site within a half-centimetre along the same gyrus may have no effect whatsoever (Ojemann, 1983, p. 193).

These findings from stimulation research provide strong support for the notion that language functions are discretely and focally represented in the left hemisphere (although a 'single' function like 'naming' can be impaired with stimulation of a number of separate sites), and that there is considerable individual variability possibly related to such individual differences as pre-operative IQ and sex.

The limitations of the electrical stimulation method are: (a) the population under study is made up of patients with often long histories of neurological disease, mainly severe epilepsy and Parkinson's disease; (b) it is not clear whether the stimulation effects neural inhibitory or excitatory activity; (c) time available for behavioural testing is limited. The major problem, however, is again one of interpretation of the findings. This is exacerbated by ignorance regarding the actual effects on neural tissue of relatively gross electrical stimulation and ignorance of the role of the surface of the cortex. It is not clear whether surface cortical structures represent 'centres' of some sort or transmission way-stations (or something else). The fact that electrical stimulation disrupts a particular function at a particular site, therefore, tells us only that that site is involved in some aspects of the function and not *how* it is involved. The contribution of electrical stimulation is comprehensively reviewed by Ojemann (1983) with valuable accompanying commentaries.

BEHAVIOURAL METHODS

Dichotic listening

Dichotic listening is a widely used behavioural technique for the investigation of hemispheric processing, and one that has been favoured in investigations of brain damaged patients. It will therefore be considered here in some detail.

The technique was developed primarily from early work by Broadbent (1954) who was among the first to observe that normal subjects tended to show a right ear advantage, preference or superiority for verbal material (Broadbent used digits as stimuli) when simultaneously presented, but different, stimuli were received at both ears. The paradigm was developed and extended to neuropsychological research primarily by Kimura (1961, 1967). Many dichotic studies have been carried out since this early work; Berlin and McNeil (1976) recently listed over 300 dichotic studies all using a variety of methodological procedures, stimulus materials, response methods, and populations. Useful recent introductions can be found in Beaumont (1983) and Code (1984a); the latter of which is particularly concerned with the application of the method with clinical populations. The popularity of the method probably has a great deal to do with its simplicity. Once a dichotic tape has been obtained or constructed (a time-consuming and labour intensive process) an investigator simply has to ensure that he or she has good quality, well-balanced, stereo playback equipment available before designing an experiment.

In essence the method involves the simultaneous presentation of different material to the separate ears of a subject via stereophonic headphones. As one item or token occurs at the left ear, a different token occurs at the right ear. A range of stimulus materials have been used, typically labelled 'verbal' (CVC words, CV syllables, digits, nonsense words, etc.) or 'non-verbal' (music, environmental sounds, tonal contours, etc.), and the general, but not unanimous, finding is that right-handed normal subjects show a right ear advantage (REA) or preference (REP) for 'verbal' stimuli (Kimura, 1961, 1967; Bryden, 1963; Shankweiler and Studdert-Kennedy, 1967; Studdert-Kennedy and Shankweiler, 1970) and a left ear advantage (LEA) or preference (LEP) for 'non-verbal' stimuli (Kimura, 1964; Curry, 1967; Knox and Kimura, 1970; Gordon, 1970; Haggard and Parkinson, 1971; Bryden, Ley, and Sugarman, 1982; Gregory, 1982).

The predominant model invoked to explain the dichotic effect is that first proposed by Kimura (1967). A contralateral and an ipsilateral auditory pathway leave the inner ear. The contralateral pathway runs to the primary auditory cortex in the temporal lobe opposite the ear, and the ipsilateral pathway travels to the primary auditory cortex in the temporal lobe on the same side as the ear (Figure 1). So although auditory stimuli entering a single ear travel to both hemispheres under normal circumstances, in the artificially induced dichotic situation the contralateral pathway is seen as inhibiting or

26

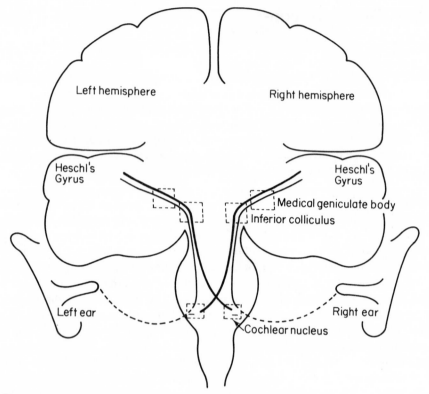

Figure 1 The contralateral and ipsilateral auditory pathways. See text for explanation.

blocking the signal travelling via the weaker ipsilateral pathway. The contralateral pathways are physiologically larger, and are seen on the Kimura model as being stronger and more efficient. The observed REA for verbal materials is explained as a function of the relative superiority of the left hemisphere for verbal processing and the LEA for non-verbal stimuli as a reflection of the relative superiority of the right hemisphere for non-verbal processing.

The ear advantage commonly observed in dichotic studies appears to be dependant upon the different phonetic or stimulus characteristics of the competing stimuli. On verbal tasks using initial stop consonants normal subjects tend to show a preference for voiceless over voiced stops, for velar place of articulation over alveolar place, and for alveolar over bilabial place of articulation (Darwin, 1974; Berlin and McNeil, 1976; Berlin and Cullen, 1977; Hayden, Kirsten, and Singh, 1979; Speaks, Carney, Niccum, and Johnson, 1981).

An REA for stops has been a more or less consistent finding, but ear advantages for normally produced vowels have not been observed. This may be because consonants are seen as being perceived linguistically and 'categorically', whereas vowels are seen as being perceived more acoustically and 'continuously' (Liberman, Cooper, Shankweiler, and Studdert-Kennedy, 1967). Darwin (1974) showed that consonant discrimination appears to be based on categorical phonetic features held in short-term memory, whereas the discrimination of vowels, which are considerably longer in duration, may be achieved on a non-linguistic acoustic basis. Interestingly, however, an REA for vowels has been obtained when white noise was added (Weiss and House, 1973), when the vowels were produced by two different sizes (synthetic) of vocal tract (Darwin, 1971), and when subjects were not aware of which of two speakers would produce a particular vowel (Haggard, 1971). Such manipulations reduce intelligibility and speed up decay. An REA is obtained because it is thought that the left ear stimulus fades or decays more rapidly in acoustic memory while the right ear stimulus is being processed, thus reducing the left ear score.

Despite the popularity of the dichotic technique in normal and clinical studies (Code, 1984a) difficulties exist with regard to the presentation of the stimuli, the methods of response employed, the test–retest reliability and the actual interpretation of the results. With regard to the use of such tests with brain damaged subjects it is extremely doubtful whether the method can be used at all as an index of hemispheric preference. This is discussed further in Chapter 7.

Many dichotic studies employ synthetic computer-generated and controlled stimuli. The advantage being that synthetic 'verbal' material can be stringently controlled for onset, offset, duration, frequency, and intensity, as well as selectively manipulated for a variety of experimental motives. Such manipulations may be concerned with staggering presentation of items, precisely specifying degree of friction, varying format transitions, etc. There are indications that some synthetic CV syllable tapes may be perceptually too difficult to be useful, especially with brain damaged subjects (Niccum, Rubens, and Speaks, 1981).

Much has been made in the literature of the mode of presentation in dichotic tasks, with some tests requiring the subject to attend to three or more rapidly presented items at each ear and report as many as are recalled. There are a number of problems with this method in the testing of aphasic patients who have reduced auditory retention. There is evidence to suggest that an increased memory load increases right ear scores (Yeni-Komshian and Gordon, 1974) thereby giving an artificially enhanced score (Bryden and Allard, 1978). One way of eliminating memory effects is to require subjects to report only a single stimulus item (Studdert-Kennedy and Shankweiler, 1970; Haggard and Parkinson, 1971; Bryden, 1978). The majority of studies with aphasic subjects have employed a single-response method for this reason. Shanks and Ryan (1976), in their aphasia study support this approach:

An ear advantage cannot be detected on trials where both stimulus items are correctly or incorrectly perceived. Analysis of trials in which only one (item) is correctly perceived focuses attention only on those items which show an ear preference and thus may be a better indicator of stimulus lateralization (p. 102).

They found that a single-response method was able to discriminate more clearly between subgroups by excluding accuracy of report from the analysis. The test–retest reliability with some tests is reported to be poor (Blumstein, Goodglass, and Tartter, 1975), with as many as 30% of normal subjects reversing ear preference on retest. In contrast, it is of significant interest to note that studies with brain damaged subjects produce good test–retest reliability figures and the simpler rhyming CVC word tests using single-report also produce good test–retest figures with both normal and brain damaged subjects (Johnson, Sommers, and Weidner, 1977; Code, 1981; Niccum et al., 1981).

Another problem which is of particular importance when comparing the results of dichotic studies is that different patterns of response may be observed depending on whether a free-recall method is employed (where subjects report as many items as they can remember), or a forced-choice method (where the subject is required to choose between one of the pairs of tokens presented). With a precued partial-report method the subject is expected to report the token or tokens at the ear specified by the experimenter. With this procedure the subject is typically tapped on the left shoulder for the left ear item, or the right shoulder for the right ear item. This method appears to reduce individual strategy variables. There is also variability between studies in the mode of response employed which further complicates comparisons of results. The response modes employed by various studies have been oral, written, and gestural. In the last method the subject points to written word or digit or a picture from a multiple-choice array. This has been particularly popular in studies with brain damaged subjects, especially those who may have severe expressive difficulties. Although there has been little systematic study in the area, the method of response would appear to be a variable which significantly affects performance.

There are other problems with the actual nature of the dichotic test used. Particular problems exist for the method which requires a subject to respond to several pairs presented in rapid succession, again, especially with brain damaged subjects who may have attentional or auditory retention problems. Such tests may introduce a number of strategy variables (Bryden, 1978). The evidence also suggests that an increased memory load increases the right ear score (Yeni-Komshian and Gordon, 1974) resulting in an 'artificially' enhanced laterality score (Bryden and Allard, 1978). One way to eliminate possible memory effects we well as a variety of possible strategy variables is to employ single pairs of stimuli (Studdert-Kennedy and Shankweiler, 1970; Bryden, 1978), and most dichotic studies with aphasic patients have used single pairs. It has also been observed that ear differences are enhanced when both stimulus items are reported and the item reported second (rather than first) is compared across ears (Satz, Aschenbach, Pattishall, and Fennell, 1965; Goodglass and Peck, 1972). Dichotic listening has been relatively widely used as a technique to investigate hemispheric preference in brain damaged populations, although the foregoing has indicated that the position of the technique in general neuropsychological research is undermined by lack of certainty regarding a number of crucial issues. With brain damaged subjects further complications emerge which are fully discussed in Chapter 7.

There are serious questions regarding the reliability and validity of the technique and although pooled group data tend to show significant differences, when individual subjects are compared it has been noted that between ear differences are as low as 2–6% (Schulhoff and Goodglass, 1969).

Hemi-field viewing

Hemi-field viewing, hemi-retinal viewing, tachistoscopic viewing or divided visual-field viewing is probably the most widely used behavioural technique in contemporary neuropsychology. The development of the technique owes much to commissurotomy research and there are a number of innovative variants that have been employed. The interested reader is recommended to White (1969) and the excellent collection edited by Beaumont (1982). The essential features of the technique are that graphic or pictorial stimuli are presented to one or both hemispheres by brief exposure (usually less than 200 milliseconds (ms)) in either the left visual field (for projection to the right hemisphere) or the right visual field (for projection to the left hemisphere) while the subject is fixating a central point on a viewing screen. This method of ensuring presentation to only a chosen hemisphere is possible because sensory information from the temporal hemi-field of the left eye and the nasal hemi-field of the right eye project via the optic nerve to the right occipital cortex, while input from the temporal hemi-field of the right eye and the nasal hemi-field of the left eye project to the left occipital cortex. Using accuracy of report or reaction times, an investigator can examine the capacity of a chosen hemisphere to process particular forms of material. Material has been back-projected from a slide projector on to a ground glass screen and presented via tachistoscope. Both unilateral and bilateral exposure have been used. In unilateral exposure stimuli are presented (usually randomly) to either the left or right visual-field; whereas in bilateral exposure stimuli are presented to both visual-fields simultaneously. Both methods have produced visual-field advantages or preferences for different types of material, although there has been much discussion as to which is the most reliable.

Hines (1972) found that a bilateral word recognition task produced a non-significant left visual-field preference which was interpreted in terms of a 'directional scanning' hypothesis where subjects recognized more words in the left visual-field due to the adoption of a left-to-right reading strategy. However, McKeever and Hulings (1971a,b), McKeever, Suberi, and Van Deventer (1972) and Hines (1972) have shown that when a central fixation digit is included for report a right visual-field preference is produced. The use of vertically presented words, rather than horizontally presented words, also appears to minimize a directional·scanning strategy (Barton, Goodglass, and Shai, 1965). However, the more natural horizontal presentation yields the expected RVF preference when controlled for fixation (McKeever and Hulings, 1971a,b; Hines, 1972) and would, *prima facie*, appear to reduce the possibility of errors on the part of aphasic patients. The use of fixation controls may induce a 'priming' effect depending on the actual nature of the fixation. There are indications that left visual-field scores can be increased for verbal material if this material is preceded by material which usually produces a right visual-field advantage (Paivio and Ernest, 1971; Kimura and Dornford, 1974; Kershner, Thomae, and Calloway, 1977) Paivio and Ernest obtained a right visual-field advantage for pictures which were preceded by the exposure of letters, but a left visual-field advantage for the pictures when they were presented before the letters. Kimura and Dornford presented letters and geometric forms to two groups and found that when forms followed the presentation of letters a significant right visual-field advantage was obtained for the forms. When forms were presented first and followed by letters, a small non-significant left visual-field advantage was obtained for forms with a significant left visual-field advantage for letters. Kershner *et al.* tested 5- to 6-year-old children on tachistoscopic tasks which used digits as verbal stimuli and either a digit or a geometric form at fixation. Results showed that the verbal fixation control produced a significant right visual-field advantage and the non-verbal control a significant left visual-field advantage.

An innovative development in the area has been the half-occluding contact lens technique (Dimond, Bures, Farrington, and Broawers, 1975; Zaidel, 1975). The method involves the subject wearing contact lenses which prevent vision in a chosen visual-field and allow stimulus material to be exposed and remain lateralized for longer periods. As a consequence standardized testing procedures have been administered to the disconnected hemispheres of commissurotomy subjects, and these studies are examined in Chapter 3.

Haptic processing

There have been few neuropsychological investigations into lateral asymmetries using the tactile modality. This is probably because haptic (tactile) studies have failed to produce reliable asymmetries and because the tactile modality does not normally function as a language modality in the way that the auditory and visual modalities do. A number of clinical tests for astereognosis (tactile agnosia) are described by Goldstein (1974) which involve palpation of objects unseen by the patient, and writing digits or letters on the fingertips in random sequence. For a 'lesion effect' to be revealed on haptic testing, it is considered necessary for there to be almost complete extinction of response from one hand on dichhaptic (simultaneous bilateral) stimulation.

Witelson (1974) employed a dichhaptic method to examine tactual asymmetries in 47 normal right-handed boys (mean age 11.6 years), which involved the dichotomous presentation of two pairs of upper case letters (one pair to each hand) with a 2-second pause between pairs. Each letter was presented for 2 seconds. Two pairs were used with a 2-second pause between them in order to introduce a memory factor, and an oral response was required in order to ensure left hemisphere mediation at some point during information processing. No differences were observed in accuracy of response using this method. Witelson suggests that although tactual letters are linguistic symbols, they are also spatial stimuli, and may consequently require right hemisphere processing. Her results, she suggests, are consistent with the hypothesis that tactually presented verbal material is initially analysed in a spatial code by the right hemisphere. However, it has been suggested that the age of the subjects might have mitigated against asymmetries being revealed as it is possible that hemispheric development may be incomplete in this age group (Oscar-Berman, Rehbein, Porfert, and Goodglass, 1978). However, as discussed earlier, recent research in developmental neuropsychology suggests that hemispheric functional superiority is established early in children. Cohen (1977) concludes that:

> most researchers assume that responses made by the whole hand can be mediated by either hemisphere, but that responses requiring fine control of individual fingers can only be mediated by the contralateral hemisphere (p. 199).

However, a recent study (Oscar-Berman *et al.*, 1978) has produced asymmetries between the palms of normal right-handed subjects using a dichhaptic stimulation method. Both palms of subjects were stimulated by writing digits, letters, and line orientations on them simultaneously. A right-hand advantage was revealed for letters, left-hand advantage for line orientations, and no differences were revealed for digits. However, the asymmetries for letters and lines appeared only on second report, and the investigators suggest that this indicates that hemispheric asymmetry only emerges when the subject's memory for tactually presented information is involved. Asymmetries were not revealed for initial perception of the material.

Lower level tactile perception of letters and words appears to be processed in such a way that asymmetries are not revealed between hands. This may be, as Witelson (1974) contends, because such stimuli require spatial as well as verbal processing. Indeed, it has been argued (Harris, 1980; Harris and Carr, 1983) that tactile processing is actually biased towards spatial–Gestalt right hemisphere processing. Harris (1980) cites the evidence from blind subjects who show a left hand superiority for individual Braille letters. Harris and Carr (1983) point out that the skin is relatively slow in discriminating the temporal and spatial aspects of stimuli compared to the visual system. They suggest that:

> underlying right-hemisphere superiority (as manifested through the left-hand advantage) is that discrimination is by touch rather than by sight (p. 71).

They conclude that:

> sensory modality interacts with functional demands in determining the hemispheric locus of processing (p. 71).

Oscar-Berman *et al.*'s (1978) findings suggest that asymmetries in haptic tasks may be revealed only when higher information-processing stages (e.g., categorization, encoding, storage, retrieval) are involved.

Lateral eye movements

A further behavioural method that has been used to some extent to investigate hemispheric involvement in cognitive processing is that of lateral eye movements (LEM's).

It is a common observation that people often gaze briefly to one side of the other of space while reflecting on a question and it has been reasoned that:

> while engaged in verbal thought, a person should visibly orient to the right, not in order to look at anything in that direction, but as an involuntary accompaniment of the cognitive process (Kinsbourne, 1974, p. 279).

Conversely, it has been argued, thought involving visuospatial reasoning should be preceded by eye movements to the left (Bakan, 1969; Bakan and Shotland, 1969; Kinsbourne, 1972, 1974; Kocel, Galin, Ornstein, and Merrin, 1972).

Kocel *et al.*, presented 16 young male and 13 young female subjects with two groups of 20 questions requiring verbal and visuospatial problem solving (e.g., 'Define the word "economics"; Solve the following arithmetic problem: $144/6 \times 4$'); spatial problem solving and musical tasks (e.g., 'There is a profile of George Washington on a quarter, which way does he face?' Hum "Row, Row, Row, Your Boat"'). The former were considered to involve left hemisphere and the latter right hemisphere processing. The procedure involved seating the subject some $4\frac{1}{2}$ feet in front of a video camera and the questions were read over an intercom. The results of this study supported the hypothesis that the cognitive demands of the question determine the direction of LEMs which indicate the activation of the contralateral hemisphere: left LEMs were associated with the 'right hemisphere' tasks and right LEMs with the 'left hemisphere' tasks.

Kinsbourne (1972) tested 20 right-handed and 20 left-handed undergraduates on 20 verbal, 20 non-verbal, and 20 visuospatial questions while the subject was seated in front of a video camera, which was hidden behind a curtain. The questioner was seated behind the subject. The direction of head movements as well as LEMs was observed. Right-handed subjects made more horizontal and right LEMs than vertical or left LEMs in the verbal condition. No differences were observed during visuospatial questioning. Head movements were generally vertical and upwards for non-verbal and visuospatial conditions in right-handers and horizontal head movements were more common during verbal questioning. For left-handers horizontal movements were more common under all conditions, but no major differences were observed in left or right horizontal LEMs or head movements. The results were interpreted to conform to the notion that for right-handers the left hemisphere is superior during verbal processing and the right hemisphere during visuospatial processing. Left-handers, however, have a more heterogeneous hemispheric organization.

The question has been raised in the literature regarding the role of stress and anxiety caused by experimenter/questioner location in LEM studies (Kinsbourne, 1974; Gur, Gur, and Harris, 1975). Apparently, when the experimenter sits behind the subject LEMs are contralateral to the hemisphere considered to be specialized for mediation of the cognitive processing engaged by the question. However, when the experimenter faces the subject the general finding is that subjects gaze consistently to either left or right irrespective of the kind of question asked (Duke, 1968; Bakan, 1969; Huang and Byrne, 1978). Gur *et al.* (1975) used both procedures with the same subjects and confirmed the findings of previous studies: LEMs emerged with the experimenter seated behind the subject and consistent eye gaze in one direction only was observed in the face-to-face condition. Gur *et al.* suggest that the face-to-face procedure arouses anxiety which causes the subject to adopt a preferred cognitive mode and hemispheric mediation. Berg and Harris (1980) in a replication and extension of this study failed to confirm the findings. They compared the two standard experimenter–location conditions with a third one. This involved the experimenter being seated behind the subject having first caused stress by making comments like 'Did you find these questions too hard?'; 'Do you expect to graduate?'; etc. No differences emerged in anxiety ratings on the standard experimental procedures but anxiety ratings were significantly higher for the stressful condition. No interaction between experimenter position or stress condition and eye movements was observed. In addition, not only was there no significant relationship between LEMs and type of question (verbal or spatial), but what relationship was observed was in the unexpected direction: right LEMs were non-significantly associated with spatial and left LEMs were non-significantly associated with verbal questioning.

The failure of replication and the uncertainty regarding the role of anxiety presents problems in interpreting the LEMs research and the role of the technique:

> All these discrepancies raise concerns about the reliability and validity of lateral eye movements as an index of hemispheric activation (Berg and Harris, 1980, p. 92).

Verbal–manual time sharing

Kinsbourne and Cook (1971) developed a verbal–manual time-sharing paradigm where a subject is required simultaneously to perform a verbal and a manual task:

If the tasks, such as right-finger tapping and verbalization, are programmed by the same hemisphere—for example the left hemisphere manual performance suffers in comparison to control conditions where right-finger tapping occurs in silence. If the two tasks are separately programmed, one by each hemisphere—for example, left-finger tapping and verbalization—no disruption in manual performance is noted compared to control conditions (left-finger tapping in silence) (Klingman and Sussman, 1983, p. 26).

The explanation for these effects is that the verbalization and right-hand activity are being mediated by the same left hemisphere and either overloading the cognitive capacity of the hemisphere or causing a conflict or time-sharing situation. During left-hand activity and verbalization no such conflict occurs; each hemisphere is responsible for a task. The interference effect of the verbal–manual time-sharing paradigm has been demonstrated in children (Kinsbourne and McMurray, 1975; Piazza, 1977) and adults (Hicks, 1973) and has provided support for the notion that children with language delay or disorder have atypical language lateralization (Hughes and Sussman, 1983). Sussman (1982) observed an atypical pattern of performance in left-handed and stuttering subjects when compared to right-handed controls using a verbal–spatial time-sharing method, and Klingman and Sussman (1983) have recently reported that some Broca's aphasic patients produce abnormal patterns of performance indicative of atypical hemispheric representation for language. These latter findings are discussed more fully in Chapter 7.

What appears to be of particular interest from the point of view of examining hemispheric capacity in brain damaged patients, is that the method should not be as susceptible to lesion effects as other behavioural methods. In view of this, and the relative simplicity of the technique (which is not dependant on the availability of complex and expensive laboratory equipment), there should be an increase in its use with brain damaged patients.

CONCLUSIONS

From the perspective of examining the role of the right hemisphere in behaviour, an isolated right hemisphere is not the same as a right hemisphere separated from its neighbour, which, in turn, is not the same as a right hemisphere with a damaged neighbour. None of these is the same as a normal brain, and there is strong evidence to indicate that there is wide individual variability in hemispheric organization related to such factors as age, sex, and handedness.

The foregoing discussion has highlighted the dominant problem in interpreting the findings of all neuropsychological research: that of establishing the quality of the data obtained from a variety of sources using a range of neurophysiological and behavioural methods. It is now clearly recognized that the findings obtained from different populations are not directly comparable, and caution should be exercised in comparing data obtained from a common population using different techniques of investigation.

The results of behavioural studies with normal and clinical populations may be flawed by a failure to control for a whole range of individual differences and individual strategies adopted for dealing with experimental tasks. In experimental studies with normal subjects it is predominantly behavioural methods which are used. These techniques mainly estimate perceptual preferences via sensory modalities, and findings cannot, therefore, be used directly to support notions concerning expressive aspects of language.

Information gained from neurophysiological investigations may be considered by some to be more reliable than the results of experiments using behavioural methods, but such investigations are overwhelmingly carried out with brain damaged patients, and it is not always clear how to interpret the data obtained from some neurophysiological techniques. Different methods of investigation provide very different information about the brain depending on the technique used. Information may refer to structural changes in neural tissue due to damage, bloodflow patterns and metabolic changes during functional activity, or changes in behaviour caused by some kind of induced temporary local or complete hemispheric 'lesion'. The technique may also provide purely superficially cortical or deeper subcortical information.

Any discussion of the role of particular regions of the brain in behaviour, such as the one undertaken in the rest of this volume, must attempt to evaluate the evidence from many directions while keeping in mind the currently recognized limitations of the source of the evidence.

Chapter Three

LINGUISTIC COMPREHENSION IN THE RIGHT HEMISPHERE

In this chapter we examine the evidence for right hemisphere comprehension of straight linguistic aspects of language in a range of clinical and normal populations. We will be concerned with those aspects of language which are most suitably dealt with by a grammatical model. Thus, those aspects of language which can be analysed in terms of phonological, syntactic, and lexical–semantic parameters are discussed. It is precisely these parameters of language which are traditionally credited with purely left hemisphere representation and it is predominantly deficits in these areas which characterize the aphasias resulting from unilateral left hemisphere damage.

There is reason to suppose that the right hemisphere's involvement in the comprehension of language is superior to its involvement in the expression of language. In fact, while most would accept the contemporary position that the right hemisphere plays a significant role in comprehension, many would contend that it has no expressive abilities at all. So we begin this chapter from the position that, first, the right hemisphere is involved in comprehension and, second, that it may have the ability to understand some aspects of language for which an underlying phonological, syntactic and/or semantic competence is required. The question we ask, therefore, is to what extent does phonological, syntactic, and lexical–semantic processing take place in the right hemisphere?

We review the evidence for linguistic comprehension in the separated right hemisphere and the isolated right hemisphere. The recent evidence for a deficit in linguistic comprehension in the unilaterally damaged right hemisphere is also examined, as well as research with the neurologically normal.

COMMISSUROTOMY

Early studies

The first commissurotomy studies begun in the early 1960s and conducted by Sperry and Gazzaniga on the Bogen–Vogel series of patients (Bogen and Vogel, 1962; Gazzaniga, Bogen, and Sperry, 1962, 1963), at first showed that the right hemisphere possessed little or no linguistic capability. However, with the introduction of new testing techniques, it began to become clear that the right hemisphere was not 'word-blind' and 'word-deaf', which had been

Geschwind's (1965a, b) interpretation of the earlier findings (Gazzaniga and Sperry, 1967; Gazzaniga, 1970; Sperry and Gazzaniga, 1967; Searleman, 1977). For instance, initial reports showed that patients (mainly N.G. and L.B.) were found to be able to retrieve a named object with their left hand from a selection of objects shielded from their view. It became clear that the right hemisphere was able to comprehend the verbal instructions given for the retrieval of such objects as a pyramid, coin, fork, tack, and pliers. The right hemisphere had to understand the commands in order for the left hand (which had no interhemispheric connection to the left hemisphere) to retrieve the objects. As well as being able to understand the meaning of such high frequency concrete nouns it was also able to demonstrate processing capability for such adjectival phrases as 'measuring instrument', 'eating utensil', and object definitions such as 'used to drive nails' and 'kept in the bank'. Also, the patients showed that they could point to objects with their left hands following the projection of printed object names (e.g., spoon, cup, pin) to the right hemisphere only via the left visual hemi-field. The right hemisphere in these patients also demonstrated that it could spell simple words like 'hat', 'how', 'dog', and 'what' when the left hand was presented with a scrambled selection of cut-out letters.

In addition this early work seemed to indicate that the right hemisphere could recognize semantic associations between words like 'shoe' and 'sock', 'cigarette' and 'ashtray', and 'hand' and 'ring'. Thus, although the early studies demonstrated a right hemisphere competence in commissurized patients for handling relatively simple concrete nouns, the indications were that syntactic processing was limited (Gazzaniga, 1970; Gazzaniga and Hillyard, 1971). It appeared, for instance, that patients were unable to respond to simple verbal commands flashed to the right hemisphere such as 'tap', 'smile', and 'frown'. Gazzaniga and Hillyard (1971) found that when a picture like that of a boy kissing a girl was projected to the right hemisphere only, N.G. and L.B. were unable to indicate which of active or passive tensed sentences 'the boy kisses the girl' or 'the girl kisses the boy' was correct. A failure of the right hemisphere to recognize future tense was also apparent where patients were unable to make the correct distinction when a picture of a girl drinking or about to drink was flashed to the right hemisphere and followed by the question, 'Which is correct? The girl is drinking or the girl will drink?' However, the right hemisphere was apparently able to process affirmatives and negatives. When a picture of a girl either sitting or not sitting was flashed to the right hemisphere the correct alternative from 'The girl is sitting' and 'The girl is not sitting' was selected almost every time. This report also stated that the right hemisphere was unable to differentiate the singular from the plural. For instance, when pictures of either one or several dogs jumping a fence were presented to the right hemisphere, the patients showed the ability to distinguish between the examiner's spoken alternatives, 'The dog jumps over the fence' and 'The dogs jump over the fence'.

In a study of right hemisphere linguistic abilities with five commissurotomy patients (N.G., L.B., A.A., C.C., R.Y.), Levy and Trevarthen (1977) found little or no evidence of a right hemisphere capacity to deal with simple semantic or phonological (rhyming) tasks. In their first experiment a strong left field–right hemisphere superiority was found for palindrome chimeras, where three short palindromes (deed, noon, sees) were divided and recombined into bilaterally presented stimuli (e.g., deon, noed, dees). The response involved pointing to one of the choice of three palindromes. When asked to respond orally subjects responded primarily to the right field–left hemisphere stimuli:

> The strong right hemisphere dominance for word matching indicates either that the four-letter monosyllabic words were being responded to as nonsense shapes without semantic content, or that the right hemisphere is dominant for the perceptual aspect of reading such words if no vocal output is required (Levy and Trevarthen, 1977, p. 110).

In their following experiment Levy and Trevarthen examined the possible role of the separated right hemisphere in semantic decoding. Chimeras were made up for bilateral presentation from the words 'lady', 'ball', and 'shoe' (e.g., lall, bady, shll) and the subject was required to point to one of three pictures representing the words. It was hypothesized that in order to perform correctly, the stimulus words had to be responded to as meaningful symbols and not simply as visual configurations. Results showed that for the vast majority of trials a right field–left hemisphere advantage was obtained. It will be recalled that earlier studies had indicated that when whole words were unilaterally projected to the right hemisphere, commissurotomized patients were able to select the appropriate picture, Levy and Trevarthen (1977, p. 112) suggest, therefore, their results indicate that:

> The apparent linguistic incompetencies of the right hemisphere for visual input cannot be attributed to an inability to derive the semantic content of words, but must, rather, be attributed at least in part, to a strong competitive predominance of the left hemisphere for such functions.

In their third chimeric study, Levy and Trevarthen examined the ability of the separated right hemisphere to perform tasks dependent upon phonological processing by requiring it to make associations between pictures of words which rhymed (e.g., rose–toes, eye–pie, bee–key). Chimeras were created where half a picture (e.g., rose) was projected to one hemisphere and another half picture (e.g., eye) to the other hemisphere in bilateral presentation. The subject's task was to point to one of three pictures which had a name which rhymed with the picture seen in the tachistoscope. Most subjects showed a highly significant left hemisphere advantage for this task. One patient, C.C. (with extensive left hemisphere pathology), did show some right hemisphere capacity on the task, but still produced a superior left hemisphere performance.

Following up these results Levy and Trevarthen unilaterally presented the same whole pictures in the left field where subjects responded by pointing to a picture of a word which rhymed with one flashed to the right hemisphere. Most subjects would not perform the task although C.C. scored 14 out of 24. No right hemisphere capability was shown either when this task was repeated but after each presentation the examiner asked, 'Does it rhyme with . . . ? Levy and Trevarthen (1977, p. 116) conclude:

> Both hemispheres have some capacities for understanding all forms of sensory input, their functional asymmetries reside predominantly in their encoding capacities which are a function of their inherent processing mechanisms. The left hemisphere can understand visual input, but is able to encode visual–imagistic representations only of a much lower level of efficiency than the right. The right hemisphere can understand spoken language and perceive basic language forms but cannot generate acoustic–verbal images. . . . Results of the rhyming objects test strongly suggest that the right hemisphere lacks a phonetic analyser that can also generate phonetic images.

These earlier observations on the linguistic capabilities of the separated right hemisphere have been extended more recently by the introduction of new techniques and a series of new patients.

More recently the sophisticated contact-lens technique discussed in Chapter 2 has been utilized by Zaidel (1976, 1977, 1978a,b) to extend knowledge further. The technique allows stimulus material to be presented to a chosen visual field and to remain lateralized for longer periods. As a consequence, standardized testing procedures for determining comprehension levels, such as the Peabody Picture Vocabulary Test, Ammon Full Range Picture Vocabulary, the Token Test, and selected subtests of the Boston and Minnesota aphasia batteries have been administered to the disconnected right hemisphere.

Zaidel (1976) produced evidence for substantial auditory language comprehension in the right hemispheres of the patients he has tested. Patients N.G. and L.B. were tested on the Peabody, Ammon's, Boston, and Minnesota tests. Results demonstrated that the separated right hemisphere has a picture vocabulary equal to or better than that of a 13-year-old child (this average is taken from the two separate scores of the two subjects, L.B. and N.G., and does not include the scores of the left hemispheractomy patient included in the study). L.B. obtained a right hemisphere MA of 16.3 and 13.5 on the Peabody and Ammon's respectively (mean 14.9) and N.G. and MA of 11.0 and 10.0 (mean 10.5) on the same two tests. The study failed to find any differences in the comprehension of object nouns and progressive verbs by the right hemisphere. Auditory comprehension was also examined on the non-redundant Token Test (Zaidel, 1977) and it was found that average scores of the right hemisphere were comparable to a 4-year-old child. This contrasts with the high mental age achieved on the Peabody and Ammon's tests. Zaidel (1977) suggests that poor performance by the right hemisphere on the Token Test could be due to a lack of a sequential short-term verbal memory capacity in the right hemisphere. He proposes that the different cognitive styles of the two hemispheres determines the way analysis of a linguistic task is carried out. The right hemisphere determines the meaning of a word by its acoustic Gestalt rather than the analysis of the word's phonetic components as is thought to be carried out by the left hemisphere. The left hemisphere may:

> store the reference in short-term memory as an abstract linguistic representation so that the features of each word are analysed serially. The right hemisphere, on the other hand, may first map the reference phrase into some nonlinguistic visual representation (say, an image) (Zaidel, 1977, p. 13).

Zaidel suggests that his results support the view that there is a qualitative difference in the linguistic comprehension capabilities of the hemispheres. He suggests that not only are the two hemispheres different in their capacity to process linguistic material, but they differ in the way in which they handle linguistic material. During comprehension the left hemisphere appears to store auditory information in terms of an abstract linguistic representation processed by categorical phonetic-feature extraction. The right hemisphere appears to analyse words in a holistic manner in terms of their auditory Gestalt and re-encodes linguistic material for short-term storage into non-linguistic visual information.

Zaidel (1978a) examined the right hemisphere abilities of L.B. and N.G. on the Carrow Test of Auditory Comprehension of Language. In this test the ability to differentiate between minimal syntactic pairs is assessed (e.g., selecting from three pictures the appropriate one which corresponds to the sentence 'She shows the girl the picture', where the two foil pictures entail a woman showing a boy a picture of a girl and a woman showing a boy a picture of a boy). The results showed that the right hemisphere of N.G. had a syntactic competence of around five years and L.B. one of more than seven years. In fact, the right hemisphere of L.B. actually performed better than the left hemisphere which Zaidel (1978) attributes to a ceiling effect.

Recent studies

A second series of commissurotomy operations carried out by Wilson (Gazzaniga, Risse, Springer, Clark, and Wilson, 1975; Wilson, Reeves, Gazzaniga, and Culver, 1977; summarized in Gazzaniga, 1983) has produced new data on the capacity of the right hemisphere in language and, because the operation currently leaves the anterior commissure intact, some insight into the nature of interhemispheric communication. A number of studies have concentrated on the remarkable right hemisphere capabilities of the single subject P.S. This right-handed boy experienced a severe series of epileptic attacks at about age two years with left temporal lobe focus. He then apparently developed normally until age 10 years when the seizures recurred. Complete sectioning of the corpus callosum was performed in 1976 (Wilson *et al.*, 1977). At age 15, within a month of surgery, it began to become apparent that P.S. had a certain degree of bilateral representation for language functions, presumably as a consequence of his early epileptic history. What is particularly remarkable, however, is that the subject's right hemisphere language capabilities appear to be developing with time since surgery.

Gazzaniga, Le Doux, and Wilson (1977) reported that P.S. at age 15 years was able to point to pictures from multiple-choice arrays depicting action verbs (e.g., sleeping, laughing, eating), which had been presented to the right hemisphere, on 10 out of 10 trials. He was able to match words that were lateralized to the right hemisphere with their opposites (e.g., girl–boy, circle–square, child–adult) on 4 out of 4 trials and score 5 out of 6 correct when required to choose a word conceptually associated with one presented to the right hemisphere (e.g., clock–time, porch–house, court–judge). He scored perfectly on a phonological rhyming task which presented words to the right hemisphere for matching with rhyming words from an array (e.g., tie–buy, rose–knows, knee–pea) and he was able to correctly spell the name of seven common objects (e.g., apple, bicycle, sheep) presented to the right hemisphere, by arranging plastic letters as well as by writing with the left hand. At least in this patient a significant syntactic, phonological, and semantic competence has been demonstrated.

The caution with which the split-brain evidence should be interpreted was referred to in Chapter 2. The indications are that the right hemisphere abilities of split-brain subjects, and P.S. in particular (who is assumed to have undergone considerable hemispheric reorganization early in life and also since surgery), cannot be generalized to the normal brain. However, the observation that this individual's right hemisphere continues to develop language processing capabilities may have significant relevant to issues concerning the recovery from aphasia following left hemisphere damage as discussed in Chapter 7.

A recent study (Sidtis, Volpe, Wilson, Rayport, and Gazzaniga, 1981) has examined further the semantic and phonetic capabilities to the right hemisphere in two patients (V.P., J.W.) from the Wilson series. V.P. is a 27-year-old right-handed female and J.W. a 26-year-old right-handed male at time of testing and both have histories of epileptic seizures.

In the semantic trials three- to five-letter high frequency nouns were presented unilaterally on a video screen under microprocessor control. The five semantic relationships examined were synonym (e.g., boat–ship), antonym (e.g., day–night), function (e.g., clock–time), superordinate category membership (e.g., lake–water), and subordinate category membership (e.g., tree–oak). Subjects were required to point to (and not name) the word related to the stimulus word by the specified rule (e.g., means the opposite) from a choice of four words with the hand homologous to the visual-field of presentation (e.g., left-field word, left-hand response). In addition, a Verbs Test was completed by V.P. and J.W. where one of six common verbs (write, play, strike, pour, drink, eat) was presented to a visual-field and the subject was required to demonstrate the meaning of the word with one of 12 objects available using the homologous hand.

Results showed that right hemisphere performance on all six tests was significantly greater than chance for both subjects, although V.P.'s right hemisphere performance was superior to J.W's. These results confirm others which have shown a right hemisphere semantic processing capacity and verb comprehension capability in the isolated right hemisphere. In this same study the phonetic processing capacity of the isolated right hemispheres of V.P. and J.W. was examined. In this experiment a CV syllable dichotic test requiring written response and a CV discrimination test where a non-dichotic binaural CV syllable was presented following dichotic presentation and on half the trials the syllable was the same (and on half different) as one of the preceding dichotic pair. Subjects responded by pointing to either 'yes' (for a match) or 'no' on response cards. This discrimination task apparently shows a left hemisphere advantage in normal subjects. A visual rhyming test was also completed by both subjects using the microprocessor–video presentation system where 24 high frequency nouns were unilaterally presented and the subjects were expected to choose a rhyming word from a multiple-choice array using the hand homotopic to the field of presentation.

The expected and now classic effects of corpus callosum section on dichotic performance were shown. Right ear scores were above normal and left ear scores were below normal performance demonstrating that the left ear stimuli are not transferred to the left hemisphere for report and the right ear stimuli are processed by the left hemisphere without the interference of the competing information from the left ear–right hemisphere–corpus callosum route. On the CV discrimination test the right hemisphere performance (matching of syllables presented to the left ear–right hemisphere with right hand response) was below chance. However, with left hand (left ear–right hemisphere) response V.P. produced a nearly perfect performance while right ear performance was below chance. On the visual rhyming test J.W's. right hemisphere performance was little better than chance (25% correct) while V.P's right hemisphere score was well above chance (75% correct). These results with two recent split-brain patients are of interest for a number of reasons. They confirm some earlier results and show that there is great variability in the cerebral organization of different individual patients, with V.P. showing a significant right hemisphere capacity for phonetic and phonological processing (forms of processing thought only to be mediated by the left hemisphere in the normal brain) and J.W. showing little or no right hemisphere phonetic processing capability. Sidtis *et at.* interpret these results to suggest that the differences between the hemispheres in language processing abilities are quantitative rather than qualitative:

performance variability reflects differences in capacity that are more obvious in some tasks (e.g., phonetic processing) than in others (e.g., semantic processing) (Sidtis *et al.*, 1981, p. 329).

Of further significant interest is the observation that V.P., like P.S., is developing and improving her right hemisphere linguistic capabilities, providing some support for the plasticity hypothesis.

We examine next comprehension in the few reports concerned with the mature isolated right hemisphere.

LEFT HEMISPHERECTOMY

Hemispherectomy describes the complete surgical removal of a cerebral hemisphere, whereas hemidecortication implies the removal of the lobes of the neocortex while leaving intact parts of the thalamus and basal ganglia (see Chapter 2). These radical procedures are usually performed on patients suffering from large and life-threatening brain tumours. One difficulty in assessing evidence from left hemispherectomy studies is that most of these patients had surgery during the first few years of life and are reported to have developed near normal language. From the perspective of making any contribution to knowledge of right hemisphere in the mature brain, therefore, it is the mature hemispherectomy patient who is the most interesting and relevant. It seems likely that the remaining right hemisphere in these two groups may process information differently. The equipotentiality controversy, and recent developments thereon, is discussed more fully in Chapter 2.

As has been observed (Coltheart, 1980a), the detail and care in examination of the language functions of some of the adult cases is disappointing. Zollinger (1935), for instance, examined language in a right-handed woman (age 43 years) who had undergone hemispherectomy and concluded that 'an elementary vocabulary was retained, which was partially increased by training' (p. 1063), but comprehension abilities are not mentioned. Other cases, however, apparently had considerable comprehension abilities. Crockett and Estridge (1951) reported a case of left hemispherectomy who could 'comply with simple commands' (p. 75) and could distinguish his left from his right hand on the day of surgery. He was also able to copy diagrams, letters, and figures but could not read and could not recognize the significance of the diagrams he had copied. No further qualitative information is given. Hillier's (1954) case was a 15-year-old boy who had two operations for glioblastoma within a year before the left hemisphere was removed. On discharge (36 days post-surgery) 'he appeared to have perfectly normal powers of comprehension of the spoken word and appeared to enjoy music considerably' (p. 720). At 27 months post-surgery the patient was said to have accurate comprehension of the spoken word and was able to read individual letters but not words (whether this was in reading aloud or not is not detailed).

The mature case described by Smith (Smith, 1966; Smith and Burkland, 1966) and examined by Zangwill (1967) has received the most attention due to the more detailed examination of neuropsychological functions. Moreover, the case is a true hemispherectomy as 'all four left cerebral lobes, limbic forebrain and basal ganglia were completely removed' (Smith, 1966, p. 467).

Examination revealed some ability to follow commands after surgery and at 6 months post-surgery the patient (E.C.) was able to reply to 'Is it snowing outside?' with 'What do you think I am? A mind reader?'. At 7 months following surgery he was able to write the word 'cow' beneath a picture of that animal. He made gains in verbal comprehension reflected in Peabody Picture Vocabulary Test scores and attention span continued to improve. The patient was able to select printed colour names on cards and correctly identified 14 out of 14 objects placed in his left hand (but not his right). Smith observes that comprehension was initially less impaired and showed greater recovery than expression. Zangwill's (1967) examination of E.C. some 18 months after the operation confirmed that the patient could read some object and colour names, but was unable to read sentences, even simple ones. He had good auditory verbal comprehension and could print his own name although he could not write the names of objects to dictation or spontaneously.

The left hemispherectomy patient would appear to have substantial language comprehension abilities which can only be accounted for by remaining brain.

UNILATERAL RIGHT HEMISPHERE DAMAGE

Early observations

Until relatively recently one of the strongest myths of neuropsychology has been that unilateral right hemisphere damage does not produce language problems. There has been a rapid increase in the number of studies of the apparent language problems of right-hemisphere-damaged subjects in just the last few years and these are discussed in detail in this section.

It was the observations of Eisenson (1962, 1964) which posed the first serious questions regarding the intactness of language following right hemisphere damage. Eisenson (1962) used a range of vocabulary and sentence completion tests to compare a right-hemisphere-damaged group (number unspecified), all of whom were right-handed with damage limited to the right hemisphere, to a control group (number also unspecified). Results indicated marked impairments in the experimental group on some tasks. Significant deficits were noted in a multiple-choice recognition vocabulary test, a sentence completion test requiring the use of abstract words for correct completion, a sentence completion test which required abstract words on some tasks and concrete words on others to correctly complete the sentences (differences between groups were greater for abstract than for concrete words).

Eisenson (1962) concluded that the right hemisphere is not devoid of language, but is involved in higher-level language processing:

> We suggest that the right hemisphere might be involved with super or extra-ordinary language function, particularly as this function calls upon the need of the individual to deal with relatively abstract established language formulations, to which he must adjust (p. 53).

The language impairment of the right-hemisphere-damaged individual is not apparent during the course of normal casual conversation, and is seldom picked up on standard aphasia tests. The subtlety of the impairment, together with the dogma of left hemisphere dominance for language, is clearly what accounts for past failures to recognize that such patients do have language deficits. Eisenson (1964) considered that the patient's problems became evident when tasks became difficult and abstract:

> Where the right-brain damaged individual can speak or formulate, in a situation of his own making, or initiate a formulation, he will do pretty well; if he only has to define words, he will define them fairly well, but really subtle and abstract meanings will escape him. He tends to become a little more concrete in his definitions. Where he has to deal with structured sentences that someone else has formulated he begins to have real difficulty. The more abstract the sentence the more difficulty the person with right-brain damage tends to show (p. 216).

More recent studies have attempted to examine more closely the nature of the deficit following right hemisphere damage, and, as with other areas of contemporary neuropsychological study, they have sought to determine the independent status of the right hemisphere deficit. Studies have concentrated on determining the linguistic level of deficit and controlling for the possible influence on poor performance of left unilateral spatial neglect, often found in right-hemisphere-damaged patients.

Lesser (1974) compared the performance of 15 right-hemisphere-damaged CVA patients, 15 left-hemisphere-damaged CVA patients, 15 normal controls, and 9 bilateral frontal leucotomy patients on syntactic, semantic, and phonological tests of comprehension. Both the semantic and phonological tests required the subject to point to a picture from a multiple-choice array of four, where one picture corresponded to the target word and the others represented either close associations (semantic test) or were phonologically similar (phonological test). The picture arrays were arranged in two columns of two. Patients were also tested on a battery of aphasia tests, the Standard Progressive Matrices and the English Picture Vocabulary Test (EPVT).

The right-hemisphere-damaged group performed significantly worse than controls on the Progressive Matrices, EPVT, and the semantic comprehension test and produced scores comparable to the normal controls on the syntactic and phonological tests. Although bilateral brain damage cannot be ruled out in the right-hemisphere-damaged group, such damage would be expected to produce significantly depressed scores on other linguistically based tests, which did not occur. Additionally, the low scores on the EPVT and semantic tests might be accounted for by a left unilateral spatial neglect, but the phonological test also employed a multiple-choice array method and scores on this test were almost as good as for the normal controls. A unilateral spatial neglect explanation on its own, cannot account for the poor performance of the right hemisphere patients on the EPVT and semantic test. Lesser (1974, p. 256) cautiously concludes that:

the tentative findings reported in this present study are not incompatible with the speculation that right hemisphere damage can interfere with the understanding of the meaning of single words, while the syntactic interpretation of sentences by the left hemisphere is relatively unaffected.

Recent studies

Hier and Kaplan (1980) tested 34 right-hemisphere-damaged subjects on a vocabulary test, a complex logico-grammatical sentence comprehension test, and a proverbs test. They found that the experimental group performed as well as normals on the vocabulary test, but some, though not all, had difficulties in comprehending logico-grammatical sentences and interpreting proverbs. These deficits, they suggest, were related to difficulties in grasping spatial and passive relationships and tended to correlate with visuospatial impairments. There was a possibility also that the comprehension deficits were related to impaired attention. However, a recent series of Italian studies have attempted to refine methods in order to control for visuospatial and attentional factors.

Cavalli, De Renzi, Faglioni, and Vitali (1981) have produced evidence that the language deficit of right-hemisphere-damaged patients may be highly specific. They tested 40 right-hemisphere-damaged patients (32 CVA, 8 tumour) and 35 controls on a range of tests. All patients were stated to be free from left unilateral neglect. Tests included the Token Test, the Reporter's Test (the expressive version of the Token Test) and a naming to description test which required the subject to provide the name of an object, animal, profession, etc., after the examiner's description. Additional tests were the word fluency test which required the subject to say as many words as possible beginning with 'P', 'F', and 'L', and a sentence anagram test where patients had to rearrange separate words on cards into appropriate sentences. The right-hemisphere-damaged group performed significantly worse than controls on only the sentence anagram test. The authors acknowledge that poor performance on this test may have been due to such general effects of brain damage as reduced attention and motivation, but point out that such factors should also impair performance on some of the other measures. The authors conclude that the patients' ability to grasp the basic syntactic rules underlying word order in the test was not markedly impaired, but:

> there are hints that when a subtle appreciation of the role played by phrases that are not essential is required, RH patients lack sensitivity for their value and proper position (Cavalli et al., 1981, p. 552).

Furthermore:

> The most common type of error was to leave the sentence unfinished or to produce sentences with unlikely meanings, either because the patient failed to perceive the key role played by some phrases in supporting the sentence

architecture, or because he did not realise that simply changing the position of a phrase would emphasize the sense of the sentence (Cavalli *et al.*, 1981, p. 553).

A series of studies of unilateral right-hemisphere-damaged subjects by Gainotti and associates (Gainotti, Caltagirone, and Miceli, 1979; Gainotti, Caltagirone, Miceli, and Masullo, 1981; Gainotti, Caltagirone, and Miceli, 1983) has been directed at investigating the relationship between an apparent selective impairment of semantic–lexical discrimination, left unilateral spatial neglect, and general mental deterioration in right-hemisphere-damaged patients. In their first study, Gainotti *et al.*, (1979) administered an auditory verbal comprehension test to 110 right-hemisphere-damaged patients and 94 controls, consisting of 20 concrete noun pictures which the subjects were required to point to from multiple-choice arrays of six pictures arranged in two columns of three. Each array was made up of the target noun, a phonemically related noun, a semantically related noun, and three unrelated foils. It was argued that the presence of left unilateral spatial neglect should have no effect on those test items where the target word appeared in the right hand column of the multiple-choice array. In addition, all patients were assessed on a general mental deterioration battery.

Results showed that the experimental group made significantly more semantic errors than the controls but that most of the errors occurred when the target word appeared in the left column in the array. This suggested strongly that most of the semantic errors were due to the presence of left unilateral neglect rather than a semantic discrimination impairment. In addition, significantly more errors were made by those subjects designated 'deteriorated' than by those classified as 'non-deteriorated'. In fact, the performance of the non-deteriorated right hemisphere group was only slightly worse than that of the controls.

In a second study, Gainotti *et al.*, (1981) were concerned to reduce further the influence of left unilateral neglect by arranging stimuli in one single vertical column and to examine more closely performance of right-hemisphere-damaged subjects on tests of phonemic discrimination and lexical–semantic reading comprehension. Fifty right-hemisphere-damaged subjects and 39 controls were administered a range of tests including the auditory verbal comprehension test that was used in the first study. In addition there was a reading comprehension test where the subject was required to read a concrete noun and then point to the appropriate picture on the vertically arranged array of six pictures made up of the same mixture of semantic, phonemic, and unrelated pictures as the auditory–verbal comprehension test. Also administered were the mental deterioration battery and a nonsense-syllable phonemic discrimination test where subjects were asked to say whether two nonsense syllables spoken by the examiner were the same or different; if different, the syllables contrasted in either voice, place, or voice and place. Non-significant differences were found between control and experimental subjects in performance on the phonemic discrimination test, supporting the notion that the right hemisphere is not involved in phonological processing. On auditory–verbal comprehension and reading comprehension tests the right-hemisphere-damaged subjects did significantly worse than the controls, but when deteriorated subjects were excluded from analysis highly significant differences in performance by controls and right-hemisphere-damaged subjects existed only for the auditory–verbal comprehension test. Differences in performance on reading comprehension just failed to reach significance. Even so, there was no significant statistical difference between mean auditory and reading comprehension errors. These results appear to support the view that the right hemisphere has a lexical–semantic function which operates better through the auditory than visual modality, and that the deficit in right-hemisphere-damaged patients is separate to unilateral spatial neglect.

In their third study, Gainotti et al., (1983) were concerned to examine whether subtle visual perception difficulties, often associated with right hemisphere damage, may have mediated to affect performance on the earlier studies employing multiple-choice arrays in testing and also to investigate the speech production of right-hemisphere-damaged patients for semantic errors. In this study 65 right-hemisphere-damaged and 74 controls were administered a confrontation naming test where errors were classified blind by judges into visual (e.g., 'ball' for 'apple'), semantic (e.g., 'peas' for 'apple') and visual–semantic ('peach' for 'apple'). Experimental subjects were also administered the mental deterioration battery. Results showed that, as with the previous studies, mentally deteriorated right-hemisphere-damaged patients made the most errors and that both visuoperceptual and lexical–semantic disorders accounted for these errors. The non-deteriorated right hemisphere patients produced mainly visual–semantic and purely semantic errors and few purely visual errors. When compared to the control group's performance the difference was significant for the visual–semantic errors and just failed to reach significance for purely semantic errors. The authors suggest that as the semantic discrimination errors produced by the non-deteriorated right-hemisphere-damaged patients were predominantly visual–semantic and purely semantic (rather than simply visual), then the significant influence of a visual perception disorder can be ruled out. The series of studies completed by Gainotti and co-workers provides further evidence that right-hemisphere-damaged patients with general mental impairment, is independent of a general cognitive deterioration and independent of left unilateral spatial neglect and visual perception deficit. In addition, the specific lexical–semantic deficit is mainly apparent when lexical access is through the auditory rather than the visual–graphic modality. The findings also confirm other observations that the right hemisphere is minimally involved in phonological processing.

Gainotti et al. (1983) suggest that a future study might examine the performance of right-hemisphere-damaged patients on a task involving the discrimination of both concrete and abstract nouns to resolve the question of whether the semantic deficit of such patients may still be due to a high level cognitive deficit. As discussed in a following section, the right hemisphere appears to be involved in the processing of concrete nouns but deficient in the processing of abstract nouns. Gainotti *et al.* predict that subjects would make more errors on discriminating concrete nouns if they had a specific and independent lexical–semantic disorder, and more errors on abstract noun discrimination if a general high level cognitive deficit underlies their difficulties with lexical–semantic discrimination.

Bishop and Byng (1984) have reported some findings obtained from brain damaged subjects on a test of semantic discrimination which, on the face of it, appear to undermine the lexical–semantic deficit hypothesis; however, there are serious methodological flaws in the study. The subjects examined by Bishop and Byng were a group of 31 subjects between 35 and 40 years post-trauma with brain damage due to penetrating gunshot wounds (17 left-hemisphere-damaged and 16 right-hemisphere-damaged). Presumably, although information is not given on ages of the subjects, brain damage occurred during the Second World War in the subjects' late teens or early twenties. In contrast, the randomly selected patients studied by Gainotti's group were CVA and tumour patients of much more recent onset and older when damage occurred. Details are not given in any of these studies, but presumably Bishop and Byng's subjects had many more focal injuries as compared to Gainotti's diffusely damaged patients. These are major differences with significantly different effects on performance (see Chapter 2). Little information is provided on severity of initial brain damage or cognitive deficit, although it is clear from the poor performance on a number of measures that many of the subjects in the Gainotti series had significant cognitive impairments. Bishop and Byng's subjects, in contrast, apparently had few cognitive deficits of any kind. Of the left-hemisphere-damaged group 10 had apparently been aphasic at time of injury, but only 3 had persisting aphasic symptoms, and only 1 was severely aphasic. Also examined by Bishop and Byng was a group of 11 left-hemisphere-damaged aphasic patients of more recent onset (details not provided), apparently with marked cognitive deficits.

Bishop and Byng's testing procedure involved presenting eight multiple-choice pictures in an oval array, where targets were presented with semantic, visual, visual–semantic, and semantically unrelated distractors. Neither a normal control group nor the large group of left- or right-hemisphere-damaged subjects produced significant errors on this test. Bishop and Byng conclude that right hemisphere damage does not produce a lexical–semantic discrimination deficit. There was also a failure to find evidence for significant semantic comprehension deficit in the large left-hemisphere-damaged group. This is in interesting contrast to the 11 aphasic patients of more recent onset and more significant brain damage. Seven of these patients produced evidence of semantic comprehension deficit and it was the three global aphasic patients who had the most problems with the test. Although seven is too small a number from which to generalize, there is evidence of lexical–semantic discrimination deficit subsequent to left hemisphere insult when brain damage is sufficiently severe actually to cause problems. The large right-hemisphere-damaged group were so apparently unaffected by their brain damage that they showed little evidence of cognitive impairment of any kind. Thus, there was no evidence of visuospatial impairment of unilateral neglect in these subjects, or any other deficits associated with right hemisphere damage. In addition, these subjects were 35 to 40 years post-onset. It is really not surprising that subjects with focal lesions of long duration show little evidence of lexical–semantic discrimination impairment when they show no disturbance of other functions! We have only to look at the performance of the large left-hemisphere-damaged group and compare them to the small aphasic group to see that significant brain damage of recent onset can produce evidence of impairment of lexical–semantic comprehension.

Before the hypothesis that right brain damage may result in a lexical–semantic discrimination deficit can be rejected, we would need to see the performance of more severely damaged patients of recent onset on the tests described by Bishop and Byng The evidence from the Gainotti series of studies lends some support to the early observations of Eisenson that right hemisphere damage can indeed cause subtle impairments in language, and it extends the tentative conclusions of Lesser that the deficit affects the semantic domain. It also suggests that while visuospatial, attentional, and generalized intellectual impairments may also mediate to exacerbate the language impairment in severe patients, a specific and independent lexical–semantic deficit can occur following right hemisphere damage.

STUDIES OF THE NORMAL BRAIN

Evidence for right hemisphere involvement in language in the normal intact brain comes primarily from the perceptual paradigms of tachistoscopic hemi-field viewing and auditory dichotic listening. Some work in lateral eye movements (LEMs) has also demonstrated right hemisphere involvement in language, but this work has concentrated on emotional aspects of language, and these are considered in Chapter 5. Likewise, dichotic studies of right hemisphere language have been directed predominantly towards investigating paralinguistic aspects of language, also discussed fully in Chapter 5. Tachistoscopic viewing has therefore been the major experimental paradigm for examining hemispheric involvement in language in normal subjects.

Right hemisphere representation of concrete/imageable words

The right hemisphere's visuospatial capacity is considered to underlie a superior involvement in visual imagery. Bakan's (1980) recent review demonstrates that evidence from studies with brain damaged and normal subjects strongly implicates the right hemisphere in a range of functions involving imagery. For instance, patients with posterior right hemisphere damage have been reported to suffer a loss of the ability to dream (Humphrey and Zangwill, 1951) and individuals suffering epileptic attacks with right hemisphere foci often report 'dreamy state' auras (Arseni and Petrovici, 1971). Lateral eye movement (LEMs) research with normal subjects also tends to show that for many tasks involving imagery, left eye movements (indicating right hemisphere activation) are more prominant (see Bakan, 1980, for review). However, the LEMs research is equivocal and Bakan (1980) has suggested that the research indicates involvement of the left hemisphere for some tasks requiring imagery. Bakan speculates that the right hemisphere has a primary role in imagery (and deals with *raw* imagery) while the left hemisphere may be involved in secondary processing (or *cooking*) of images. He suggests that the right hemisphere:

> mediates the making of pictures in the head or images in other modalities. It is crucial for the production of *raw* imagery. This basic ability to produce images is what gets lost after certain right hemisphere brain injury. . . . This raw imagery may appear spontaneously under certain conditions as sleep, muscular relaxation, free association, mind-wandering, and under the influence of certain drugs . . . At times when the hemispheres are in good communication, there may be processing or *cooking* of the raw right hemisphere imagery by the left hemisphere. The left hemisphere may request that images be constructed for help in the solution of problems posed in visuo-spatial tasks . . . or the left hemisphere may take hold of raw imagery from dream recall or day dreaming, and bring to bear on it some form of logical analytic, or reality-orientated processing . . . in some imagery is neither localizable in the right or left hemisphere. Components of imagery exist in both (Bakan, 1980, p. 50).

Words can be contrasted on an abstract/concrete and imageable/non-imageable dimension (Paivio, 1971; Richardson, 1975) and there are high correlations between concrete and imageable on the one hand and abstract and non-imageable words on the other. An area which has received attention, particularly from studies with normal subjects and studies of patients with deep dyslexia (discussed in more detail in Chapter 7), has been the extent of the contribution made by the right hemisphere to the mediation of concrete and imageable words. Thus, the general finding appears to be that words which are concrete as opposed to abstract and are more easily imaged or visualized have representation in a right hemisphere lexicon whereas words which are abstract and non-imageable do not appear to have right hemisphere representation in the normal brain. However, Patterson and Besner (1984) have recently concluded that only 5 out of 18 published studies have found a significant Imageability × VHF interaction.

Ellis and Sheppard (1974) employed a bilateral tachistoscopic method where a concrete word was presented to one visual-field and an abstract word to the other, either side of a central fixation digit. Subjects were required to report orally the words that they saw. Although abstract words produced a significant right visual-field–left hemisphere advantage, concrete words did not. Ellis and Sheppard suggest that these results indicate direct right hemisphere lexical access for concrete words via imagery and indirect left hemisphere processing of abstract words via a phonological route. Hines (1976, 1977) also examined visual-field advantages for concrete and abstract words in normal subjects using bilateral presentation with a central fixation digit and oral report. Results showed a significant right visual-field–left hemisphere superiority for abstract but not concrete nouns. As noted by Bradshaw (1980) and on page 29 of this volume, the results of tachistoscopic studies which use bilateral presentation may be contaminated by left-to-right scanning artifacts.

Marcel and Patterson (1979) employed unilateral presentation, however, and a backward masking technique. They found that highly imageable words presented to the left visual-field were reported more accurately than words low in imageability. They also suggest that words which are high in imageability access a right hemisphere lexicon via a direct non-phonological imageable route.

Day (1977) conducted a series of three experiments using vertically arranged and unilaterally presented letter strings in a lexical decision reaction time task. In Experiment 1, 14 right-handed, normal, male and female subjects were tested on concrete and abstract nouns matched for concreteness ratings, word length, and frequency. The non-words were pronounceable strings of letters made up by altering a single letter in each of the words used as stimuli. Results showed a right visual-field superiority for speed of response to abstract nouns but no differences between fields for speed of response to concrete nouns.

> These findings suggest that lexical entries representing abstract nouns are accessed more efficiently in the left hemisphere, whereas lexical entries representing concrete nouns are accessed equally efficiently by both hemispheres (Day, 1977, p. 521).

Day's (1977) experiments 2 and 3 examined the ability of the normal right hemisphere in 16 male and female right-handed subjects to recognize semantic associations between the words that it knows. In Experiment 2 subjects were required to decide whether a unilaterally presented concrete or abstract word belonged or did not belong to a previously foveally presented superordinate semantic category (e.g., animal–horse; animal–rock). Results showed that abstract nouns are recognized as instances of superordinate categories when presented to the right visual-field, but that reaction times for recognizing that concrete nouns do or do not belong to a particular superordinate category do not differ as a function of visual-field presentation. Despite the indication that the normal right hemisphere is capable of making word associations, Day points out that the foveally presented category word (exposed for 1 second) may have activated or primed various semantic associations in the left hemisphere which passed via interhemispheric transfer to the right hemisphere.

In the follow-up Experiment 3, Day presented the superordinate category word and test word simultaneously to 16 male and female normal right-handed subjects. Category words were presented foveally and vertically and concrete and abstract test words were presented unilaterally and vertically in one or other visual field. Results replicated those obtained in Experiment 2, and thus provide further confirmation that the right hemisphere is able to make semantic associations between concrete nouns but not abstract nouns. Day also comments that a number of predominantly female subjects actually showed a left visual-field reaction-time advantage for abstract nouns, consistent with the view that females are more likely to enjoy bilateral representation for language than males.

Day's (1977) series of careful experiments appear to provide reliable support for the right hemisphere imageability hypothesis. However, there is evidence which questions the findings of some studies, recently reviewed by Bradshaw (1980) and Lambert (1982). Gross (1972) obtained a right visual-field advantage for pairs of concrete nouns presented unilaterally where the subject had to make a decision on whether the two nouns belonged to the same category. Bradshaw and Gates (1978) found no support for right hemisphere processing of highly imageable concrete words in a study which unilaterally presented high or low frequency, abstract or concrete words. A right visual-field advantage was found for all classes. Lambert (1982) points out that the findings of the early bilateral word recognition studies are explainable in terms of failure to control for contaminating variables. In contrast, Bradshaw (1980) implies that the use of an 'unnatural' vertical presentation of words should reduce the probability of holistic, non-phonological recognition of concrete words by the right hemisphere. Day's results, for instance, might actually have underestimated the capability of the right hemisphere to process imageable, concrete words.

Although a number of studies have indicated that words which are high in imageability and concrete can access a right hemisphere lexicon via a non-phonological route, there has been a marked failure of replication. Many of the difficulties stem from the failure to iron out the methodological problems currently inherent in studies employing the tachistoscopic hemi-field viewing method with normal subjects. In later chapters we examine the contribution of evidence from clinical studies to the right hemisphere imageability hypothesis.

Dichotic studies have produced little evidence for right hemisphere processing of strict linguistic aspects of language in normal subjects, although those which have examined ear advantages, and by implication hemispheric advantages, for paralinguistic features of language are discussed in Chapter 5. Two recent dichotic studies have provided some support for the right hemisphere imageability hypothesis. McFarland, McFarland, Bain, and Ashton (1978) examined ear differences for abstract and concrete words. Abstract and concrete words were presented to one ear and a competing stimulus to the other ear. A right ear advantage for abstract words and no ear advantage for concrete words emerged when the competing stimulus was speech. Kelly and

Orton (1979) observed similar levels of recall accuracy for both ears when high imageability words were presented to the left ear and low imageability words were presented to the right ear. A right ear advantage was observed, however, when low imageability words were presented to the left ear and high imageability words were directed to the right ear. Although there would appear to be some support from dichotic studies for the view that the right hemisphere is able to process concrete words which are highly imageable via the auditory as well as the visual system, Lambert and Beaumont (1982) suggest that Kelly and Orton's findings do not support the right hemisphere hypothesis. They point out that the small ear differences observed when high imageability words were presented to the left ear and contrasted with low imageability words to the right ear is accounted for by a combination of a normal right ear advantage for verbal material and an expected advantage for high imageability words cancelling each other out.

Right hemisphere reading

Reading is the other major modality of linguistic comprehension and we will examine below what is currently understood of the right hemisphere's reading abilities in normal subjects. Our understanding in this area has been much advanced by recent development in research into deep dyslexia and related reading problems following unilateral left hemisphere damage, and these developments are considered in Chapter 7. As stated earlier, our appreciation of right hemisphere linguistic processing in normal subjects has come mainly from tachistoscopic studies employing graphic material.

We have seen earlier in this chapter that the normal right hemisphere (in right-handed male subjects at least) appears to be unable to derive phonology from print. It was shown that this finding from studies with normal subjects is supported by the commissurotomy work, the hemispherectomy/ hemidecortication investigations, and is also clear from studies of deep dyslexia to be discussed later.

The *dual-coding* model of reading holds that two distinct processing mechanisms underlie normal reading: these are direct visual processing resulting in direct lexical access, and phonological processing. It may be noted at this point that direct lexical access requires holistic–Gestalt processing whereas access via an indirect phonological route is dependent upon grapheme-to-phoneme transformation rules which require segmental–analytic processing. Our current understanding of the cognitive processing capabilities of the hemispheres would suggest that direct lexical access is better dealt with by the right hemisphere and phonological processing by the left hemisphere.

Right hemisphere processing of ideographic script

The distinct kana and kanji orthographies of Japanese have received a good deal of attention in hemispheric investigations of reading because they provide a unique opportunity to examine both direct lexical access and phonological access in the same individual (see Sasanuma, 1980, for review). Kana is a phonetic, syllabic script where each written symbol respresents a spoken syllable and kanji is ideographic, like Chinese script, where a single written character represents a lexical morpheme. A kanji character does not contain information on how the word should be pronounced and an unknown word written in kanji is both incomprehensible and unpronounceable. The same word written in kana could be pronounced, if not understood (Colt-heart, 1980a). In Japanese orthography contentives are usually represented by kanji characters (although they can be represented by phonetic kana characters) whereas function words and grammatical morphemes such as inflectional verb endings can only be represented by kana characters. Thus kanji characters are appreciated holistically and do not require phonological decoding in order to determine meaning. Segmental phonological analysis is required for kana characters. As the holistic–analytic mode hypothesis of hemispheric processing predicts, findings from studies which have directed attention to the contribution of the two hemispheres in the processing of these two distinct scripts strongly suggest that the right hemisphere is superior in its abilities to deal with holistic kanji script while the left hemisphere is better able to deal with segmental kana script (Coltheart, 1980a). Thus, visual-field studies with normal Japanese subjects have shown that verbal report is more accurate for kana symbols (and words involving more than one kanji charac-ter) when presented to the left hemisphere via the right visual-field (Hatta, 1977; Sasanuma, Itoh, Mori, and Kobayashi, 1977), whereas verbal report for single kanji characters is more accurate when presented to the right hemisphere (Hatta, 1977). These experimental results from normal subjects are supported by research with left-hemisphere-damaged Japanese aphasic and adult acquired dyslexia patients which shows that for many there is a selective impairment in kana processing but a relative preservation of kanji processing (Sasanuma, 1980).

It has been pointed out (Lambert, 1982) that ideographic kanji are visuospatially quite complex while linguistically quite simple, which may account for a good deal of the right hemisphere advantage. Additionally, the task demands of some experiments may also contribute to the reported left visual-field advantage for kanji characters. Some studies have found, for instance, that when two kanji characters are combined in one visual field, thereby making the task more linguistically complex, a right visual-field advantage is observed (Kershner and Jeng, 1972; Hatta, 1978; Tzeng, Hung, and Cotton, 1979).

To summarize thus far, there is evidence for a right hemisphere reading system which employs direct lexical access and is incapable of phonological access. In addition, evidence from studies with Japanese readers tends to support the hypothesis that the right hemisphere has special abilities, related to its visuospatial processing powers, which enable it to deal with graphic material which requires holistic, direct visual access.

CONCLUSIONS

Early work indicated that the separated right hemisphere was able to comprehend common concrete nouns, adjectival phrases, object definitional phrases, and could spell simple short words and recognize semantic associations between common nouns. Little syntactic processing was demonstrated in the right hemisphere in the earlier work: it could not process active versus passive, future tenses, or distinguish singular from plural but could differentiate affirmatives and negatives. Little or no phonological ability has been demonstrated in the right hemisphere of commisurotomy patients. Later work showed that the right hemisphere had substantial auditory comprehension abilities as demonstrated by its performance on standard tests. It had a vocabulary equivalent to a 13-year-old child and auditory comprehension for longer complex phrases was comparable to a 4-year-old child. In addition, syntactic competence above the 5-year-old level was demonstrated. Auditory comprehension of non-redundant instructions was found to be at around the 4-year-old level, perhaps due to poor short-term auditory verbal memory in the right hemisphere.

Recent studies on new commissurotomy patients have confirmed some early findings. Excluding data obtained from patients P.S. and V.P., who most clearly demonstrate bilateral representation, right hemisphere processing of such semantic operations as the ability to differentiate synonyms, antonyms, function, and superordinate and subordinate category membership have been demonstrated, as well as comprehension of common verbs. In addition, the earlier observations that the separated right hemisphere possessed little or no facility for processing phonological and phonetic information has been confirmed by the recent studies, although questioned by some (Patterson and Besner, 1984). Moreover, some individual patients possess considerable right hemisphere phonetic and phonological processing capacities. The most remarkable observation from the recent Wilson series is that for some patients with bilateral representation, the right hemisphere is capable of increasing its linguistic competence with the passage of time. However, there is substantial disagreement regarding the linguistic capabilities of the right hemisphere, even among those intimately involved in the commissurotomy studies (for detailed argument see Gazzaniga, 1983; Levy, 1983; Zaidel, 1983), and on the relevance of findings for normal brains. The sparse information on adult left hemispherectomy and hemidecortication patients indicates considerable auditory comprehension abilities including understanding of verbal commands. Reading abilities have been reported to be poor, with some individuals only able to read single letters, but others having the capacity to read common object and colour names, but not even simple sentences. Some simple spelling ability has also been reported.

Recent studies with patients who have suffered unilateral right hemisphere damage have suggested deficits consistent with the notion that the intact right hemisphere is involved in auditory and visually mediated comprehension dependent on lexical–semantic processing. However, methodological issues need to be ironed out in order to demonstrate that the deficit is independent of other right hemisphere deficits. The major finding from studies with normal subjects is that the right hemisphere is capable of comprehending words which are high frequency, highly imageable, and more concrete than abstract, and of processing semantic associations between such words. The indications are that such linguistic material accessed the right hemisphere via a non-phonological visual route. This work also indicates that the right hemisphere reading system is capable of dealing with high frequency, imageable, concrete words, and studies of Japanese kanji and kana scripts support the view that the right hemisphere employs an holistic–Gestalt mode for direct lexical access.

We must again at this point reiterate the difficulties inherent in comparing the data available from the range of populations studied. The problems of replication and methodology plague experimental studies with normal subjects using behavioural techniques, producing few unequivocal results. Although findings from commissurotomy studies stand up to some scrutiny, such findings, as we have seen, cannot be generalized to normal populations directly, mainly because of the past neurological histories of the subjects. Significant variability can be observed in the right hemisphere performance of individual split-brain patients (Gazzaniga, Volpe, Smylie, Wilson, and LeDoux, 1979). This variability is demonstrated by the contrast in the range of scores obtained by Zaidel's (1976) subjects on the Peabody Test (range in Ma = 11.0 to 16.3) and by Gazzaniga's subjects P.S. and J.H. The subject P.S. has remarkable right hemisphere skills whereas it has not been possible to show any language abilities of any kind in the right hemisphere of J.H. The same is true for hemispherectomy/hemidecortication subjects. In addition, the poor quality of reportage in many of the hemispherectomy cases makes interpretation precarious. In contrast, studies of the unilaterally right-hemisphere-damaged, but previously neurologically normal, appear to have ironed-out many of the methodological problems and the way seems clear towards determining whether such patients can present with a specific lexical–semantic comprehension deficit. A further dimension is added to our enquiry when we consider the retained abilities of the unilaterally left-hemisphere-damaged patient in a later chapter.

Taking the *weight* of evidence examined in this chapter, there can be little doubt that the right hemisphere is involved in formal linguistic aspects of language comprehension. The exact nature and extent of this involvement is to be determined, but current understanding provides some support for a qualitatively different right hemisphere linguistic competence. Many workers in the field feel that the qualitative differences between the processing modes of the hemispheres can be appreciated on an holistic–analytic dimension and that right hemisphere involvement in linguistic comprehension is a reflection of its holistic–Gestalt mode of cognitive information processing. However, the variability in the evidence requires our caution.

Chapter Four

THE ROLE OF THE RIGHT HEMISPHERE IN THE PRODUCTION AND EXPRESSION OF LANGUAGE

Our faculty of speech is invariably cited as the supreme achievement of nature. Starting with the observations of Broca, the notion that this function (as well as most other worthwhile functions) was controlled exclusively by the left hemisphere became the very foundation of the dominance model and lent support to the ultimate dogma that consciousness itself was an exclusively left hemisphere concern.

In this chapter we examine the scattered but compelling evidence which has revolutionized our notions regarding the lowly status of the 'mute' right hemisphere. Interestingly, all the evidence comes from clinical studies, but before we start to look at these, we examine Hughlings Jackson's (1874) propositional–non-propositional distinction in language. Jackson's hypothesis really represents the only developed model which predicts a right hemisphere capability for speech production. Following the discussion of speech production we look at the right hemisphere's role in expression of language through writing.

THE PROPOSITIONALITY DIMENSION

It was Jackson's (1874) view that speech is either propositional and the product of the left hemisphere or non-propositional or automatic and mediated by both hemispheres:

> the right hemisphere is the one for the most automatic use of words, and the left the one in which automatic use of words merges into voluntary use of words— into speech (Jackson, 1874, pp. 81–82).

Jackson's conception of this duality in language, unique when initially proposed, was formed following his observations on the language disorders of brain damaged individuals. This notion, that there were two kinds of spoken language which could be distinguished on a propositionality dimension, was very different to the monistic theory of language held at that time (Goldman-Eisler, 1968). A number of writers since Jackson have utilized propositionality in discussions of language, extending, reformulating in some cases, and providing support for neurophysiological and behavioural characterizations of the notion (Head, 1926; Goldstein, 1948; Goldman-Eisler, 1968; Luria, 1970; Van Lancker, 1972, 1975). Goldstein, for instance, differentiates abstract (volitional, propositional, and rational) from concrete (automatic, emotional) language and Head talks of the superior, voluntary, and symbolic aspects of language in contrast to the inferior, automatic, and non-symbolic. Some, like Head, Goldstein, and Luria, have extended the idea to include cognitive functioning in general, and not just language.

Van Lancker (1972) differentiates between propositional and non-propositional language as follows:

> Propositional language behaviour includes all newly-created, original, novel sentences; automatic language encompasses conventional greetings, overused and overlearned expressions . . . pause fillers such as 'you know' and 'well', certain idioms, swearing and other emotional language, perhaps stereotyped questions and answers, commands, and so on (p. 25).

Van Lancker suggests that non-propositional language is situation–context dependent, stimulus-bound, low in semantic content, and involves highly familiar, overlearned, high frequency utterances. An important feature of the propositional–non-propositional distinction is that the same word or series of words can act propositionally or non-propositionally. What constitutes a propositional utterance is not a combination of certain words, which by themselves are meaningless, but underlying propositionalization or predication. A proposition always says something about something. As Luria (1970) puts it, it is a thought 'embodied in a sentence' (p. 188), and, he suggests, the fundamental unit of speech. A propositional utterance is a newly minted statement, unique from any other. This statement might be 100% unique in respect to all other utterances produced by an individual or only 1% unique. Whichever, uniqueness is an important hallmark of propositional language. A propositional utterance therefore expresses a unique predicate or statement, itself the product of a voluntary, intentional cognitive act. However, there is no clear and unambiguous distinction between emotional or automatic utterances and propositional utterances. For instance, the words 'yes' and 'no' are propositions if used appropriately to indicate positive or negative response to a question, but non-propositional if used automatically and inappropriately by a severely aphasic individual. A great deal of the speech that we use can be viewed as non-propositional. Clichés like 'it's always the same', ready-made phrases such as 'you know what I mean' are obvious examples. However, what for one individual is an overused phrase is for another a recently discovered and unique one. For example, in scientific literature such phrases as 'theoretical underpinning', 'the more or less consistent finding' and 'recent studies have shown that' are probably used regularly, automatically, and maybe relatively non-propositionally by some individuals. For others, however, such phrases would be novel and unusual. Some examples of the most obvious kinds of non-propositional utterances are shown in Table 1. This is not meant to represent an exhaustive or exclusive list. Not only are there

Table 1   Some Examples of None-propositional Language
(the non-propositionality of which probably varies between individuals and contexts)

Serial–automatic speech (e.g., counting, days of week, months of year, recited arithmetic tables)
Singing, recitation of overfamiliar verses and rhymes
Swearing, expletives, coprolalic, and emotional utterances
Conventional social greetings (e.g., good morning, good night, thank you, excuse me, nice day)
Conversational fillers (e.g., you know, sort of)
Overused phrases, idioms, clichés, and stereotyped expressions

probably individual differences but the propositional–non-propositional dimension would appear to operate as a continuum rather than as a strict dichotomy (Van Lancker, 1972). Thus, while speaking, an individual will produce utterances with varying degrees of underlying propositionalization; some utterances will be highly propositional, some completely automatic or emotional and non-propositional, and others falling somewhere between the two extremes of the continuum.

One implication of Jackson's conception is that the two distinct forms of language will require different information-processing routes to find expression. The non-propositional route will not involve the same number or quality of linguistic stages as the route required for a propositional utterance. An important hallmark of automatic, non-propositional utterances is that they are invariant and appear to be structured and produced holistically—they do not have 'dissoluble structure', as Van Lancker has put it. She cites Weinreich (1969) who called non-propositional language 'transformationally defective', and she points out that meaningful linguistic analysis is probably impossible as 'to structurally analyze, say, an idiom or other frozen expression—to vary it in some way, is to use it propositionally' (p. 28). On the model it is propositionalization itself which has left hemisphere representation, not necessarily the individual segments or words which make up an utterance. Thus, on this view two utterances made up of the same sequence of words can have either exclusively left hemisphere or bilateral representation, depending on whether propositionalization underlies the utterance or not.

In most of the remainder of this chapter we draw heavily on Jackson's idea as we ask to what extent the right hemisphere is involved in speech production and how best to characterize any involvement.

RIGHT HEMISPHERE SPEECH PRODUCTION: THE NEUROPHYSIOLOGICAL EVIDENCE

There are indications that the right hemisphere is capable of 'vocalization' from the classic electrical stimulation studies of Penfield and Roberts (1959).

They were concerned to determine those areas of the cortex where stimulation caused language disturbance to guide surgical intervention for patients with focal epilepsy. Vocalization of an unspecified, sustained vowel cry 'which at times may have a consonant component' (p. 120), was produced by stimulation of an area of either cortical hemisphere. This area is the precentral (and, to some extent, postcentral) gyri (Rolandic region) responsible for lips, jaw, and tongue of both hemispheres and the supplementary motor areas of both hemispheres. These observations confirm that neuromuscular control of articulation and phonation are bilaterally represented on the motor and sensory strips anterior and posterior to the central sulcus, and that a bilateral lesion is required for a permanent upper motor neurone dysarthria. However, to put the bilaterally obtainable 'vocalization' of stimulation in perspective, it is probably as closely related to propositional speech as a similarly obtained leg or arm jerk would be to tap dancing. They also reported that stimulation of the Rolandic and supplementary motor areas on the right can produce speech arrest, hesitation, repetition, and verbal perseveration. But in one or two patients (with retained ability to speak) naming problems were observed.

More recent investigations using electrical stimulation have also produced little evidence for right hemisphere speech (see Ojemann, 1983, for review). Apparently, the ability to mimic single orofacial movements is altered with stimulation of face motor cortex, often with arrest of speech, but not with stimulation outside motor cortex. Changes in mimicry of sequential oral movements, alterations in short-term verbal memory and reading ability are sometimes, but very rarely, caused by right hemisphere stimulation. A recent stimulation study (Andy and Bhatnagar, 1984) has produced positive evidence for right hemisphere speech production. Data were obtained from three patients, two of whom had intractable seizures in the right temporal lobe while the other had a history of seizure originating in the temporo-orbito-frontal lobes. All three showed left hemisphere speech production processing on sodium amytal testing. The seizures in these patients had developed following head injuries (two patients) and clipping of an aneurysm (one patient) occurring during adulthood. This study used naming and reading tasks presented on slides. The kinds of interference with speech production which have been observed in other stimulation studies of the right hemisphere were noted by Andy and Bhatnagar, but impairments of naming with intact speech were also observed. One patient produced naming errors with stimulation of the right superior temporal lobe, another patient produced naming errors following stimulation of the superior parietal and superior temporal lobes. Naming errors occurred for the other patient with stimulation of the Sylvian fissure border between the superior temporal and premotor cortex. Errors in naming in these patients occurred on from 40% to 50% of trials. The question remains as to how to interpret these data. The authors themselves do not offer much in the way of explanation, except to state that the findings support the idea that the right hemisphere has some latent linguistic abilities. Why patients who have sustained right hemisphere damage in adulthood, and suffer from intractable epilepsy as a result, should show an impairment in naming with electrical interference of the right hemisphere is not a question we can even attempt to answer usefully with our current knowledge. Maybe the stimulation was transmitted to the left hemisphere.

Using the Wada technique of intracarotid injection of sodium amytal, Milner, Branch, and Rasmussen (1968) showed that of 48 right-handed neurological cases, 43 had left hemisphere speech representation and 5 (10%) had right hemisphere representation. The authors point out that this figure of 10% is not in agreement with the literature concerned with aphasia associated with right hemisphere lesions in right-handed people, and,

> it seems most unlikely that the figure of 10% obtained in the present study represents an accurate estimate of the proportion of right-handers in the normal population who are right-hemisphere dominant for speech. There may, however, he more such cases than is generally realized (p. 370).

So although this study suggests right hemisphere speech production in 10% of right-handed individuals, it must be pointed out again that the population tested were neurological patients, many with epilepsy, a large proportion of whom may have made hemispheric shifts for speech processing. Milner and her associates (Milner, Branch, and Rasmussen, 1966; Milner, 1974) have produced findings for left-handed subjects which support the suggestion of separate hemispheric representation for propositional and non-propositional speech. Following right-sided injection of 9 out of 17 left-handed subjects with bilateral representation for speech, 7 made errors in automatic–serial speech (reciting the days of the week and counting forwards and backwards) but not in propositional naming tasks. Following left side injection, errors occurred in naming but not in automatic speech. For the other 2 subjects naming was impaired with right-sided injection and automatic speech errors occurred with left-sided injection. In certain circumstances then—whether as a result of early brain damage or as a general property of left-handers with bilateral representation for speech, propositional and non-propositional speech may be lateralized to separate hemispheres. The more recently introduced regional cerebral bloodflow (rCBF) technique developed by Lassen and associates (Olesen, Paulson, and Lassen, 1971; Ingvar and Schwartz, 1974; Larsen, Skinhoj, and Lassen, 1978; Lassen, Ingvar, and Skinhoj, 1978; Skinhoj and Larsen, 1980), has produced some data which can be interpreted to support Jackson's views on the hemispheric representation of non-propositional speech.

Larsen et al. (1978) examined bloodflow during serial speech in 18 right-handed subjects with no apparent neurological deficits. They found no significant overall difference between left hemisphere and right hemisphere measurements during automatic speech. Moreover, they found no significant activation of Broca's area, but an increase in flow in the upper premotor and sensorimotor mouth areas in both hemispheres, as well as in the auditory area of the temporal lobes. Furthermore, activity in the right hemisphere during automatic speech appears to be more diffuse and widespread than in the left hemisphere (Skinhoj and Larsen, 1980).

Bearing in mind the limitations of the rCBF technique (see Chapter 2) this would seem to indicate bilateral representations for non-propositional speech. Moreover, it suggests a more diffuse right hemisphere representation compared to the more focally organized left hemisphere capacity, lending some support to the diffuse/focal dichotomy (Semmes, 1968; see Chapter 1)—at least at the level of the cortex.

The technique does not tell us anything about deep-brain structures and it is not possible to gauge the hemispheric representation of more propositional speech from these studies. All the work does, with any degree of certainty, is to confirm previous findings concerning right hemisphere contributions to neuromuscular activity, including articulation and phonation.

PATHOLOGICAL REITERATIVE UTTERANCES: SPEECH FROM THE RIGHT HEMISPHERE?

Jackson's idea of a dimension of propositionality in language was born out of his observations on the recurrent utterances and other stereotyped expressions of aphasic patients. Recurrent utterances, he proposed, are non-propositional and the product of the right hemisphere. The value of recurrent utterances from an investigatory standpoint is that the utterance often stands alone, uncontaminated by other confounding variables: the patient with such an utterance is usually unable, in the early stages, to utter anything other than this stereotyped expression.

A recurrent utterance (RU) is an utterance made up of either recognizable words or collections of speech sounds which do not make up recognizable words, which some aphasic patients produce either every time they attempt speech, or just sometimes when they attempt speech (Code, 1982a). In severe cases, the impression the observer gets is that the patient makes no attempt to suppress the utterance, being apparently completely unaware of the pragmatic–situational inappropriateness of the utterance. In less severe cases, the patient is clearly aware that the utterance is being produced, without intention on his or her part, presumably in place of an intended utterance. This is typically accompanied by great struggle and frustration in an effort to suppress the emergence of the utterance (Jackson, 1874, 1879; Alajouanine, 1956; Critchley, 1970; Code, 1982a).

These utterances have fascinated aphasiologists ever since Jackson first drew attention to them, and a number of terms have been used to describe them. Jackson (1874) coined the terms 'recurrent utterance' and 'recurring utterance', but 'verbal stereotypy' (Alajouanine, 1956), 'verbal automatism', and 'speech automatism' are also in current use. As well as these, the terms 'monophasia' to indicate a one-word recurrent utterance (Critchley, 1970), and 'word embolism' occur occasionally in the literature. Descriptions used to characterize the essential nature of the real-word variety include Jackson's

(1874) 'formula speech', 'ready-made speech', 'stock utterances' and 'barrel organisms', as well as the more contemporary 'pre-packed speech' (Marshall, 1977). At a more poetic level, Jackson refers to these expressions as 'the rags and tatters of the patient's speech' and Alajouanine (1956) describes a typical one as 'an insignificant spar remaining from the shipwreck of speech'; even more colourful is Critchley's (1970) characterization of a patient's utterance which 'overruns the garden of his speech like a weed'.

Jackson (1874) delineated a basic classification of four types of recurrent utterance; a fragment of jargon, a single word, a phrase, and 'yes' or 'no' or both occurring together. According to Critchley (1970), Henschen (1922) writing in German analysed 100 cases of recurrent utterance from records where only one word was involved. Of these patients 63 had the utterance 'yes' or 'no', with the remaining 37 being so diverse as to defy any classification. Critchley suggests that when a recurrent utterance is something other than 'yes' or 'no' it is usually an unusual and unexpected expression, and although many are made up of recognizable words 'as the patient uses it there is no such attached significance; it might just as well be any other word, or a piece of nonsense, or a grunt' (p. 190). He suggests that any linguistic analysis of these 'pseudo-semantemes', as he calls them, is pointless for this reason.

Alajouanine (1956) conducted a study over time of 317 cases of aphasia, 30 (9.4%) of whom presented with a recurrent utterance. He describes four stages in the evolution of a recurrent utterance which do not necessarily follow the same order in different individuals. During the first stage, although the unconsciously and involuntarily produced expression remains phonemically the same, a gradually developing expressive intonation emerges, which leads on to the next stage where the patient demonstrates the reassertion of consciousness and awareness of his or her attempts to check the emergence of the utterance. A fluctuating stage comes next, where the original expression becomes less persistent and is replaced by a new recurrent utterance. Gradually propositional language reappears, which is a sign that the utterance is breaking up, and finally the utterance disappears and agrammatism emerges. This represents the classic picture of the evolution of recovering Broca's aphasia. Critchley (1970) describes a similar developmental process. However, there has been no systematic investigation of the validity of such a pattern in the evolution of such expressions.

Alajouanine identifies two basic types: those with linguistic meaning and those without. Of the latter he describes iterative stereotypies which are usually one repeated syllable, and organized stereotypies which are several syllables long. He notes that the meaningful utterances are either one-word or repeated one-word utterances. He observes also that nearly all those patients who present with the meaningless type of recurrent utterance present also with severe apraxia. In addition, Alajouanine suggests that patients are unaware that they are producing an inappropriate utterance in the early stages, and he notes that the expressions are pronounced in a perfectly acceptable manner with no sign of the apraxia of speech which emerges with recovery.

It is clear from the literature and clinical observation that the prominent characteristic of these utterances is their repetitive nature (Broca, 1861; Alajouanine, 1956; Critchley, 1970). Thus Broca's patient LeBorgne, who has come down in aphasia history with the name 'Tan' as this was one of his recurrent utterances, used this expression repetitively. Critchley gives the following examples of repetitive recurrent utterances ('zu zu', 'watty watty', 'tara tara', 'yes yes yes', and states that repetition is common, if not the rule.

Patients seem to become very adept at varying the prosodic features of their utterance to signify meaning. Intonation, stress, and rate appear to be used to great effect. Critchley describes a patient who 'by altering the melody of his speech . . . was able to utilize his words ("on the booze") with such success as to make them express his immediate desires or signify assent, negation or dismissal' (p. 206). De Bleser and Poeck (1985) have recently reported a perceptual analysis of the spontaneously produced intonation contours of 9 patients with non-meaningful CV syllable recurrent utterances. Variation in intonation was present in only half of the subjects indicating that intact prosody in such patients is not as widespread as was thought and may be more related to the impression of the listener. No instrumental work has been done on the survival of prosody in recurrent utterances and no studies of the prosody of real-word recurrent utterances of any kind have been carried out. Recurrent utterances appear to be overwhelmingly associated with Broca's aphasia (Alajouanine, 1956; Code, 1982a). Views on the underlying neuroanatomical damage responsible for Broca's aphasia have undergone radical change in the past decade, mainly due to the work of Mohr and his colleagues (Mohr, 1973; Mohr et al., 1978; Mohr, 1976). This work has identified two separate conditions which are traditionally included under the term 'Broca's aphasia'. Through autopsy and other localizing information on a number of cases, plus a retrospective review of a large hospital population and a close examination of cases from the literature, Mohr has found that a lesion restricted to Broca's area (the third frontal convolution) does not produce the severe and persisting motor aphasia associated with the syndrome. A lesion of this area, originally identified by Broca, produces only a paroxysmal disorder. There is no persisting articulatory (apraxic) or language difficulty and most patients usually recover in a week or so with any remaining impairments being minimal and difficult to detect. In contrast, the lesion which produces the classical picture of Broca's aphasia is due to a much larger lesion 'involving most of the territory of the area of supply of the upper division of the left middle-cerebral artery' (Mohr, 1976, p. 230). This area includes the operculum, the third frontal convolution, the anterior parietal region, the insula and both sides of the central Rolandic fissure. Infarction usually extends deeply into the underlying white matter. The syndrome produced by this larger lesion is that traditionally called 'Broca's aphasia', characterized by a severe and persisting apraxia of speech. There is either mutism (at its most severe) or recurrent utterance with the later emergence of agrammatism and severe associated reading and writing problems. Mohr (1973, 1976) in fact suggests that the term 'Broca's aphasia' be used for the rapidly recovering form and the term 'operculum syndrome' be used for the persisting syndrome traditionally referred to as Broca's aphasia. Recurrent utterances appear to be associated with the operculum syndrome.

The importance of subcortical white matter, including the insula, in the operculum syndrome has been recently verified by Blunk, de Bleser, Willmes, and Zeumer (1981) using CT scan examination of traditional Broca's aphasic patients. Moreover, they split their patients into a global and Broca's group and found that those globally affected patients with recurrent utterances had large lesions including frontal white matter like their Broca's patients. However, global patients without recurrent utterances had a more posterior lesion pattern. This would indicate that recurrent utterance result from larger anterior lesions encompassing those areas described by Mohr.

A recent CT scan study presents convincing evidence that recurrent utterances only occur in patients with damage to the basal ganglia (Brunner, Kornhuber, Seemuller, Sugar, and Wallesch, 1982). This study examined 40 right-handed aphasic patients, 26 of whom had basal ganglia damage. Recurrent utterances only occurred in patients with basal ganglia and cortical involvement, but not in patients with only basal ganglia involvement or only cortical involvement. In other words recurrent utterances occur only in patients with both left cortical and basal ganglia damage. Furthermore, of the 12 patients with recurrent utterances, 9 had anterior and posterior damage involving the basal ganglia and 3 had just anterior lesions (mainly Broca's area) including the basal ganglia. This would suggest that the smallest lesion required to cause a recurrent utterance is an anterior lesion including the basal ganglia. These observations also indicate that any involvement in the production of recurrent utterances by left posterior mechanisms is therefore ruled out.

Do either real-word recurrent utterances (RWRUs) or non-meaningful recurrent utterances (NMRUs) represent non-propositional right hemisphere speech? The results of analysis of a mixture of 97 RWRUs and NMRUs indicate that there are some linguistic grounds for distinguishing the two types (Code, 1982a). Table 2 shows the list of RUs from this study. Both the frequency of occurrence and the range of phonemes utilized in RWRUs is similar to normal English, but not in NMRUs. There is a progressive reversal in the ratio of consonants to vowels from normal English through RWRUs to NMRUs. In addition, there are differences from normal English in manner of articulation for both types, which is most marked in NMRUs. Both types use a predominance of plosives with a reduction in nasals, affricates, and sonarants. Phoneme combinations in both types adhere to the phonotactic constraints of the language (i.e., 'foreign' phonemic combinations are not observed). Furthermore, RWRUs do not break the syntactic rules of the language.

RWRUs are made up of high frequency one- or two-syllable words with 'I' being the most common, and initial words are usually what would be classed as stressed content words. Interestingly, it seems to be possible to classify most RWRUs into a number of distinct groups, of which a pronoun + verb

Table 2 The Real-Word and Non-Meaningful Recurrent Utterances Collected by Code (1982a)

Complete List of Real Word Recurrent Utterances

alright	I think one two	pardon for you
away away away	I said	Parrot (proper name)
BBC	It's a pity pity pity	piano
because	I want to	Wednesday
Bill Bill	I want to	Percy's died
Billy Billy	I want to one two one two	sister sister
bloody hell	I try one two and I can't	sister
Bloody hell bugger	and I want to	so and so
down	John	so so
I'm a stone	milk	better better
I bin to town	money	somewhere somewhere
fuck fuck fuck	no	three three
fuck off	no	time a time
fucking fucking fucking hell	now wait a minute wait a	tingaling
cor blimey	minute wait a minute	today
funny thing funny thing	off	two two two
goody goody	oh boy	washing machine
I can't	oh you bugger	sewing machine
I can't	oil	well I know
I can talk	factory	yep
I can try	policeman	thing
I can talk and I try	on the corner	thingy
I did not hear	paper and pencil	yes yes yes
I told you		you can't

Complete List of 29 Non-Meaningful Recurrent Utterances (those in curly brackets are from the same two subjects)

/æbɪ dæbɪ/	/pi pi/
/də də də/	/es es es/
/də də də/	/bi bi bi/
/də də də/	/bəu bəu bəu/
/də də də/	/səta səta/
/tu tu tu uuuu/	/wi wi wi/
/du du du də du/	/ɪs/
/nə nə nə/	/nəusi nəusi nəu nəu nəu/
/ini ini/	/kɪ kɪ kɪ kɑ/
/əubɑbrɜ/	/əzez əzez/
/əubɑprɜ/	/bi bi/
/ibi ibi/	/eɪ weɪ eɪ weɪ wi wi wi weɪ mmm
/hɒlətəuz/	eɪ weɪ weɪ weɪ/
/tɑ tɑ/	/dɪ dɪ dɪ/
/si si/	/kɑ/

and an expletive/slang type are the most common and interesting. All 11 expletive RUs reported by Code (1982a) were produced by male patients. A large proportion of the RWRUs (more than 30%), however, did not fall into neat groups with even superficial semantic or pragmatic content. Patients sometimes have more than one RU. When this is the case their RUs are usually phonologically, syntactically, and semantically related to each other and RWRUs and NMRUs are rarely, if ever, mixed. The results of this analysis (Code, 1982a) suggest that RUs carry the hallmarks of non-propositional speech. Some of the groups identified—expletives, serials—are fairly obviously non-propositional. They are invariantly produced, being phonemically and syntactically identical each time they are uttered, at least until they begin to break up in recovering patients. But what of the other classifiable RUs? As RWRUs are composed of identifiable lexical items arranged in acceptable syntactic strings, does this mean that the utterances had some genuine propositional and pragmatic function at some time in their evolution? Proper names in the list all referred to close relatives, mainly husbands, and were maybe produced propositionally the first time they were uttered.

The pronoun + verb type of RWRU is probably the strongest contender for propositionality, although these, like the other groups, are produced invariantly and cannot be related to the illocutionary intent of the speaker. Moreover, the fact that such a large number of patients produced utterances of this semantically and pragmatically restricted type (with three examples of 'I want to . . .', for instance) would also suggest that an individual has little voluntary control over the linguistic content of the RU that he or she ends up with. This completely unexpected and previously not described group of RWRUs (the largest identifiable group in the sample) are of particular interest from the point of view of the right hemisphere hypothesis. The impression that these usually half-finished, very personal ('I' is often the first word) utterances evoke is of an emotionally highly charged request or statement. Research examined in Chapter 5 again indicates significant right hemisphere involvement in emotional behaviour and emotional language. Why so many recurrent utterances should belong to this intriguing semantically and pragmatically restricted group is a mystery, however. Such utterances may reflect very personal emotional outbursts at initial attempts to communicate following failure to activate speech production mechanisms due to severe apraxia of speech. However, there are suggestions in the earlier literature that the meaning of a RWRU is related to the activities being pursued by the patient at the time of his or her stroke (see Code, 1982b, for discussion of notions on the origins of recurrent utterances).

There would appear to be little difficulty in describing most examples of recurrent utterances as non-propositional, automatic, emotional or ready-made speech. The data provide grounds to suppose that the two types of recurrent utterance are linguistically distinct. Although the two types are clearly unrelated at a syntactic and semantic level—NMRUs having no semantic or syntactic form—the evidence indicates that they are distinguishable on phonological grounds also. It seems unlikely that NMRUs are simply random combinations of speech sounds which do not happen to form real words. The frequency, distribution, and range of phonemes in recurrent utterances are significantly different in the two types. It may be the case that linguistic mediation is not involved at all in the production of recurrent utterances, as has been suggested (Code, 1983a; de Blesser and Poeck, 1983). This argument, interestingly, may hold more for RWRUs than for NMRUs. From what we know of the 'linguistic' structure of RWRUs and the role of the right hemisphere in the processing of non-propositional language and emotion, we are almost forced to consider that input for RWRUs (at least for the initial production of the utterance) comes straight from non-linguistic levels concerned with the communication of moods, desires, and emotions. The very paucity of substantial content in NMRUs, however, provides few real clues as to their origin.

Right hemisphere processing appears to be heavily implicated in the production of RWRUs. They are non-propositional and either emotionally charged phrases or expletives or serial–automatic in nature for the most part, and they appear to be holistically produced. In fact, RWRUs fit very well the conception of right hemisphere speech capabilities put forward by Levy and Trevarthen (1977) when they suggest that:

> the articulations of which the right hemisphere may be capable are probably formed as motor Gestalts, and are not constructed analytically from phoneme—elicited articulemes as many linguists would claim to be necessary for speaking (p. 116).

Some support for this comes from a study which subjected a temporal-lobe epileptic patient to delayed auditory feedback (DAF) during the production of his *ictal speech automatism* (Chase, Cullen, Niedermeyer, Stark, and Blumer, 1967), a type of pathological reiterative utterance occurring in epilepsy, discussed later in this chapter. The patient showed none of the usual DAF effects on speech during his production of the emotional and automatic utterances (increased amplitude and pitch, reduced rate of utterance—'artificial stuttering'), which would have indicated closed-loop auditory feedback control of his speech production (Code, 1984b). The experimenters took this to mean that the patient's speech was under open-loop control—the entire utterance was being produced as if it were a single whole rather than segmentally. The suggestion that aphasic patients are unconscious of their RUs, at least in the early stages of evolution (Alajouanine, 1956), indicates that they are literally 'automatic', produced in a pre-programmed open-loop manner as a 'motor Gestalt'.

A further aspect of recurrent utterances which implicates the right hemisphere is that past clinical observation suggests that prosodic features of recurrent utterances function normally. That is to say, individuals are apparently able to signify some meaning through the use of prosodic features. This would indicate right hemisphere involvement, as the research cited in Chapter 5 would suggest that right hemisphere mechanisms play a prime role in processing such aspects of communication. Just how intact prosodic features are in a patient with a RWRU, however, is not known as there has been no research into this area.

When we turn to NMRUs, however, we find that although the utterances are clearly non-propositional, they have insufficient 'linguistic' structure to allow us to implicate the right hemisphere. They do not appear to be produced holistically; there are no 'words' which might implicate emotional or non-propositional right hemisphere processing, and prosody is also impaired. In fact, NMRUs appear more to be produced segmentally and sequentially. NMRUs are not arbitrary CV syllable concatenations but are utterances governed by some phonological constraints. Only high frequency, motorically easy phones taken from the phonetic inventory of the speaker's natural language are combined in such a way as not to break the phonotactic constraints of the language: those segments which might be seen as being on top of the pile of the phonetic inventory. There appears to be a 'simplification' process underlying the statistical distribution of phonemes. It is the articulatory or motorically easier phones which are retained, with an increase in vowels and a corresponding decrease in consonant articulations, and a reduction in range and length of utterance. The initial production of NMRUs may therefore have been by a severely compromised left hemisphere phonological system without any right hemisphere—subcortical input.

THE RIGHT HEMISPHERE AND THE SUBCORTICAL CONNECTION: A SPECIAL RELATIONSHIP?

Starting with the observations by Penfield and Roberts (1959) on the role of the thalamus in language, and gaining impetus from the development of more sophisticated techniques of investigation, there is now acceptance that discussion in the past has concentrated too much on the mere 'bark' of the cortex, especially where speech production is concerned. While the electrical stimulation technique is not without its shortcomings, it is relevant to note that Penfield and Roberts (1959) and others since have shown that spontaneous utterances have never been evoked from cortical sites in either hemisphere. However, words and phrases have been evoked from other, deep-brain sites. Areas which have received the most attention in recent years are the thalamus, the limbic system, and the basal ganglia.

Penfield and Roberts considered that the thalamus plays a significant role in language as a centre for integration between anterior and posterior speech centres, and described the intimate pathways that connect the thalamus with Broca's, Wernicke's, and the supplementary motor area. Ojemann (1976), Jonas (1982), and Kent (1984) have recently reviewed the research on the role of the thalamus in language. This work shows that spontaneous lesions of the left hemisphere of the thalamus can produce a usually transitory aphasia characterized mainly by naming errors and verbal perseveration and also with syntactic problems, paraphasia, and jargon. Writing is also often affected but comprehension is usually intact. Surgically performed stereotaxic lesions in the thalamus for the relief of dyskinesia in Parkinson's disease produce similar problems in more than a third of cases, but again the difficulties are mostly transitory. Words and phrases have been evoked from the thalamus using electrical stimulation. Ojemann (1976) describes one elderly female patient who produced the spontaneous utterances 'that's goofy', 'twinky', 'you just made the shuck go' and 'shucks once in a while'. Another patient produced the utterance 'fish'. Some utterances were apparently produced when the patient was instructed specifically not to speak.

Lamendella (1977) has recently conducted an extremely comprehensive survey of the contribution of the limbic system to human communication, emphasizing that this complex network of cortical and subcortical neural structures of the forebrain has been ignored for too long in neuropsychology. This is probably due to the enormous complexity of the system which is, as yet, still little understood even by neurophysiologists with a specialized interest in its function. Lamendella draws attention to the social and communicative role of the system and states that it is 'the obvious candidate for the level of brain activity likely to be responsible for the bulk of non-propositional human communication' (p. 159). The limbic system seems to be 'a general information system with a wide range of functional responsibilities including a major role in emotion' (p. 175). In all mammals the limbic system is involved in producing the observable automatic signals of rage, surprise, fear, alarm, etc., and this is also the case for human beings. This involvement in communicative behaviour extends to those signals concerned with the regulation of social interaction such as expressions of dominance, submission, aggression, friendship, and male–female and mother–infant interactions. Lamendella refers to the system as:

> the 'homebase' for communication functions in primates even though both higher and lower levels of brain organization are involved in the overall behaviour complex in which limbic activity plays the dominant role' (p. 188).

It is suggested that the right hemisphere has a special relationship with affective subsystems of the limbic system which the left hemisphere does not enjoy. The manifestations of limbic communicative functions is observable in certain clinical populations, some of which may be relevant to the origins of RUs. In temporal lobe epilepsy it is regions of the limbic system which 'trigger' the seizure characterized by emotional auras and various kinds of oral behaviour as well as the ictal speech automatisms discussed later in this chapter.

Gilles de la Tourette's syndrome is an affliction which comes on usually before 13 years of age (mean 7 years), and although there is no conclusive proof that it is even a neurological disorder, the symptoms present 'limbic features'*. Males outnumber females by three or four to one (Shapiro, Shapiro and Wayne, 1972) and about 37% of those with the syndrome are either left-handed or of mixed handedness. EEG abnormalities are found in most cases (Sweet, Soloman, Wayne, Shapiro, and Shapiro, 1973). The main characteristics of the syndrome are various forms of involuntarily produced facial and body tics, grunts, barks and, after several years, automatic utterances which are usually coprolalic (utterances of an obscene and sexual nature) and sometimes echolalic. Patients are aware that they are producing these utterances but unable to suppress them, especially at times of stress (Sweet et al., 1973). There are clear parallels between these utterances and expletive recurrent utterances. Also of interest with respect to a possible relationship between RUs and the coprolalia of these patients is the fact that all expletives reported by Code (1982a) were produced by male patients. Lamendella considers that these vocalizations and coprolalia originate at the level of the limbic system.

Lamendella goes on to support the propositional–non-propositional dimension in speech and suggests that the latter may be processed in the limbic system, the thalamus, basal ganglia or midbrain, and this is why such utterances are spared following left hemisphere damage. In addition, he suggests that speech with emotional content from normal speakers, such as expletives, actually originates in the limbic system because of its affective responsibilities and that these utterances have referential meaning. Such utterances relieve affective pressures in the speaker and evoke limbic responses in the hearer.

> Emotionally charged, vulgar, or obscene speech represents, not just an interaction between the limbic system and linguistic systems, but the interconnection of the two. Emotional speech results from limbic functions that have found linguistic expression, speech that while phonologically structured and possessing propositional content finds its major role in the expression of affect. [Moreover] where a strong emotional content (positive or negative) is associated with components of the propositional message, the speaker may select words or constructions that are emotionally charged in that they have a special 'tie-in' to the limbic system, perhaps via the right hemisphere. (Lamendella, 1977, p. 213).

It is Lamendella's conception then, that the right hemisphere has a mediating role between the linguistically propositional left hemisphere and the limbic system during emotional expression. Although there is a great deal of supposition in Lamendella's thesis, it does suggest a logical explanation for some aspects of RWRUs. It suggests, firstly, that although RUs are non-propositional and automatic, the emotional ones may have been voluntary expressions the first time they were uttered, and secondly, that these utterances have their origins in the limbic system via a special interconnection between the limbic system and the cortical right hemisphere. Assuming that

* Note that others specify basal ganglia lesions (Darley, Aronson, and Brown, 1975; Kent, 1984).

the limbic system has no linguistic or phonetic programming capability, but is simply the motivational force behind the utterance, then the right hemisphere, through its capacity to provide a motor Gestalt, controls the actual motor speech activity of the phono-articulatory mechanisms.

The subcortical neuronal masses which make up the basal ganglia have been shown to be heavily involved in speech production. As mentioned earlier, CT studies suggest that a lesion in the basal ganglia (in addition to cortical damage) is necessary for the emergence of a recurrent utterance (Bruner, Kornhuber, Seemuller, Sugar, and Wallesch, 1982), and basal ganglia lesioning is implicated in various disturbances of speech production and several forms of pathological reiterative utterance (Darley, Aronson, and Brown, 1975; Kornhuber, 1977; Kent, 1984). In fact Kornhuber (1977) has proposed that the basal ganglia plays a central role in speech production and has characterized its function as that of a motor programme generator. Similarly, Kent (1984) has recently queried whether damage to basal ganglia structures 'impairs a person's ability to generate motor programs, so that those residual motor programs spared by the lesions are repeated inflexibly' (p. 317). Brunner *et al.* (1982, p. 297) suggest also that pathological reiterative speech, like recurrent utterance 'is the result of defective programming of motor speech sequences giving way for an inadequate, disinhibited, invariate subrouting which is called up unintentionally'. In fact, this group suggest that Broca's area, the supplementary motor area, and the subcortical basal ganglia complex in the left brain appear to form a multiple-representation functional system for speech production. Damage to one component produces transient aphasic symptoms, suggesting compensation by the other two, whereas damage to more than one component produces a more extensive and lasting deficit.

Pallilalia is a type of pathological reiterative utterance occurring in Parkinson's disease due to basal ganglia damage (Boller, Albert, and Denes, 1975; Darley, Aronson, and Brown, 1975; Marshall, 1977; LaPointe and Horner, 1981) and there are similarities between this disorder and recurrent utterances in aphasia. The fundamental characteristic of the disorder is the tendency for the patient to repeat words and phrases during speech. LaPointe and Horner (1981, p. 36) give examples from the patient that they studied (e.g., 'from the gods to *fortell, fortell, fortell*'; in the air *they act, they act, they act* like'; '*let me, let me* keep a little of this wedding cake'). It is also apparent that propositional speech is most vulnerable and that words beginning with stops, nasals, and affricates are more susceptible to reiteration than words starting with glides, fricatives, and vowels. These utterances may be reiterated many times until the patient runs out of breath and the disorder has been characterized as a failure to inhibit unwanted speech (LaPointe and Horner, 1981). However, Marshall (1977) has suggested that pallilalia may be syntactically conditioned.

Recurrent utterances are observed in patients with extensive left hemisphere cortical and basal ganglia damage, and it is the basal ganglia damage which causes the impairment of new motor programme generation. The reiterated production of the RWRU would appear to be undertaken by a right hemisphere deprived of input to and from the basal ganglia, but enjoying an unimpaired interaction with the limbic system. It may be that the origins of emotional-expletive RWRUs are explainable by reference to limbic system—right hemisphere interaction and that other automatic RWRUs (yes/no, serial numbers) have their origin in other, subcortical, mechanisms such as the thalamus and basal ganglia, and find expression via a right hemisphere route. NMRUs, on the other hand, could conceivably be the product of a severely compromised left hemisphere language system deprived of basal ganglia programme generation capabilities or of a right hemisphere with impaired right hemisphere—limbic system interconnections (Code, 1983a). Much of this is highly speculative of course. Testing such a characterization might involve rCBF investigations which compare the cortical involvement of the two hemispheres in the production of the two types of recurrent utterance in different patients. The effects of DAF on the production of the two types could also be compared. If disruption in the fluent production of the recurrent utterance is produced under DAF, then one might conclude that the individual is utilizing open-loop control. If, on the other hand, the utterance is relatively unaffected by the DAF, then one could conclude that the patient has minimal control over the production of the utterance. Such holistic, closed-loop control of the production of the utterance might indicate right hemisphere processing.

We turn next to a type of reiterative utterance which has direct bearing on the issue of right hemisphere speech production, the propositional–nonpropositional dimension in expressive speech, as well as the neuroanatomical origins of RUs in aphasia. These are the ictal speech automatisms (ISAs) produced by patients suffering from anterior temporal lobe epilepsy. During focal epileptic seizures originating in the temporal lobe in such patients, several forms of language disturbance typically occur: a temporary paroxysmal aphasia of which the patient is usually aware subsequent to the attack, and speech automatisms made up of recognizable words which appear to be 'linguistically correct' and for which the patient is amnesic following the attack (Serafetinides and Falconer, 1963; Falconer, 1967). It is the second of these disturbances which is of particular interest. Serafetinides and Falconer identified several relevant types of ISA: recurrent utterances, where the patient produces a repeated phrase (e.g., 'that is right, that is right', 'I must go, I must go'); irrelevant utterances which appear to be almost conversational although out of context; talking during the attack about a totally irrelevant topic; emotional utterances which may be related to an emotional and often frightening hallucinatory experience, where the patient appears to be talking to someone intent on doing him or her harm.

Serafetinides and Falconer conclude from their study of 100 patients that while the paroxysmal aphasia is predominantly associated with abnormal EEG findings over the left hemisphere, ISAs occur slightly more often with abnormal EEG findings over the right hemisphere than the left hemisphere at a ratio of about 6 : 5. This result is in general agreement with those reported by Hecaen and Angelergues (1960) who found that in 32 cases of ISA, 13 had the EEG focus over the right hemisphere, 11 over the left hemisphere, and in 8 it was not possible to decide. A more recent study (Kawai and Ohashi, 1975) reported on the EEG focus in 34 patients. While all those patients with paroxysmal aphasia had focuses over the left hemisphere ($N = 13$), of the 13 patients who produced ISAs during their seizure, 10 had right hemisphere focuses and only 3 left hemisphere focuses. To summarize briefly this section on non-propositional speech, pathological reiterative utterances of various types, and the interactions between right cortical hemisphere and subcortical structures, a fundamental conclusion must be that the right hemisphere is involved in the production of certain kinds of non-propositional speech, perhaps in particular neurophysiological circumstances. We return to this in the conclusions to this chapter.

In the next section we return to the split-brain studies to ask what evidence they have produced for right hemisphere speech production.

SPEECH PRODUCTION IN THE SEPARATED RIGHT HEMISPHERE

There have been a number of reports of right hemisphere speech production in commissurized patients but these have usually been explained away in terms of cross-cueing or pre-existing bilateral representation for speech processing. cross-cueing is the term used to describe the behavioural strategies that a split-brain patient might use during experiments to circumvent the effects of corpus callosum sectioning to allow interhemispheric communication (Gazzaniga, 1970; Gazzaniga and LeDoux, 1978; see Chapter 2). As Gazzaniga and LeDoux (1978, p. 158) have put it, we can observe 'mental system right, looking at the behaviour of mental system left, and through the behavioural cueing strategies, the two systems communicate'. For example, during an experiment aimed at assessing right hemisphere speech production capability, the right hemisphere, which knows the correct answer to a test item but is unable to express it, 'informs' the left hemisphere through external non-verbal strategies and cues. The left hemisphere then produces the spoken answer. This gives the superficial impression that the right hemisphere, which had been presented with the task, has produced the spoken response. Some indications of a speech production capability in the separated right hemisphere come from early studies by Butler and Norsell (1968), Milner and Taylor (1970), Levy, Nebes, and Sperry (1971), Levy and Trevarthen (1973) and from reports on the recent Wilson series of studies by Gazzaniga and colleagues (Gazzaniga, 1977; Gazzaniga, LeDoux, and Wilson, 1977; Gazzaniga, Volpe, Smylie, Wilson, and LeDoux, 1979; Sidtis, Volpe, Wilson, Rayport, and Gazzaniga, 1981; Gazzaniga, Smylie, Baynes, Hirst, and McCleary, 1984).

Early reports

Butler and Norsell (1968) reported possible right hemisphere speech in a split-brain patient using a precursor of the contact-lens method which allowed sustained exposure of material to one hemisphere. The subject was fitted with special spectacles which allowed this sustained exposure and which were so arranged that if the subject deviated from fixation the exposure ceased. The subject was able to name words, letters, and numbers presented to the left visual-field, including the words 'clap', 'cup', and 'six'. In naming left visual-field stimuli the subject usually needed much longer exposure and time after exposure than he did for right visual-field stimuli. Butler and Norsell suggest that the long exposure time and latency before response may be necessary to overcome left hemisphere inhibition of right hemisphere competence. It has been suggested, on the contrary, that the long exposure and response time was used for cross-cueing (Searleman, 1977), and Gazzaniga (1970) suggests that a strategy where the subject fixates some feet beyond the screen would cause the image to fall within the right visual-field without switching off exposure, thereby becoming available to both hemispheres.

Milner and Taylor's (1970) study (cited by Searleman, 1977) suggested that split-brain subjects could indicate orally whether or not they had been touched either once or twice on the left hand (indicating right hemisphere speech as the information is assumed not to pass to the left hemisphere). This observation, however, has been explained by reference to the possibility that subcortical ipsilateral connections between the left hand and left hemisphere could have provided the left hemisphere with the information necessary to make the oral response (Searleman, 1977). The left hands of Levy et al.'s (1971) two subjects were presented with two to three plastic letters out of view and were aksed to arrange them to make a word. One of the subjects was able to complete the task successfully, but was unable to say what the words were. In a second task the subject's left hand was presented with letters already arranged into words and asked either to say the word or to write it with the left hand. On some trials he was instructed to write first and then say the word, while on others he was required to say the word and then write it. The subject was able to say 5 out of 10 words, but 'in no instance could he vocally designate the correct word unless he had written it first' (p. 52). Levy et al. suggest that it is the left hemisphere which is producing the oral response because it is benefiting from bilateral kinaesthetic feedback from the left hand during the initial writing of the word. The inability of the subject to name the letters in the first task is attributed to a weaker and entirely contralateral tactile system accomplishing the task, rather than the ipsilateraly represented kinaesthetic system the subject used in word discrimination.

Recent studies

We examine below the reports by Gazzaniga and associates on the right hemisphere speech production capabilities of the subjects P.S. and V.P. As was mentioned in Chapter 3, these patients appear to enjoy bilateral representation for language comprehension as a function of early left hemisphere damage. What is particularly remarkable, however, is that both subjects have developed an apparent right hemisphere speech production capability since surgery—a capability which was not present prior to surgery. For P.S. there was a complete inability to name words or pictures presented to the right hemisphere during the first 18 post-operative months. However, between 26 and 36 months post-operation there was a remarkable increase in naming ability on these tasks, to the extent that the right hemisphere was performing at the same 100% level as the left on picture naming and 85% on three- or four-letter word identification. On a homophone task, where one of a pair of homophones was presented unilaterally and vertically to one visual-field on each trial (e.g., coat or cote, roll or rowl), he was able to name both homophones, but unable to spell the non-word homophone presented to the right hemisphere. Remarkable as this developing ability in the right hemisphere of P.S. is, perhaps the most interesting result from the Gazzaniga *et al.* (1979) study is performance on description of complex scenes exposed to the right hemisphere. Some of the responses are shown in Table 3 (from Gazzaniga *et al.*, 1979, p. 810). What is of particular interest is that not only is P.S. able to name accurately most of the pictures, but then goes on to produce a vivid description which bears little relation to the actual picture. For example, for the 'man with gun' scene, the picture depicted only a young man pointing a revolver. P.S. elaborates on the basic scene 'Gun . . . hold-up . . . he has a gun and is holding up a bank teller, a counter separates them' (p. 810). With regard to the performance of P.S. on complex scenes Gazzaniga *et al.* (1979, p. 812) comment:

> On these left visual field trials he emits a word or two that identifies the dominant activity of the scene but which seems to establish the context for a

Table 3 Examples of Verbal Response to Complex Pictures by P.S. (From Gazzaniga, Volpe, Smylie, Wilson, and LeDoux (1979) 'Plasticity in speech organization following commissurotomy'. *Brain*, **102**, 805–815. *Reproduced by permission of Oxford University Press.*)

Right Hemisphere Stimulus	*Verbal Response*
(A piece of) layer cake	'Cake . . . it was a whole vanilla cake with chocolate icing, silverware is there too.'
Exploding firecracker	'Smoke . . . coming out of a chimney, it's a small house.'
Man shearing sheep	'Man . . . he is walking through the woods.'
Couple dancing	'Some guys . . . working on building together.'
Man with a gun	'Gun . . .hold up . . . he has a gun and is holding up a bank teller, a counter separates them.'
Left Hemisphere Stimulus	*Verbal Response*
Christmas tree	'A Christmas tree standing alone.'
Fat man, sweating	'Man . . . big and fat.'
Man with gun	'Guy with a gun.'

subsequent, seemingly unrelated response. These verbal responses bear little relation to the exposed slide, but remain a plausible use of the ejaculated single word response. Furthermore, once he has emitted the initial single word, he tends not to ignore this choice and insists that the subsequent description identified the essence of the exposed slide (pp. 812–813).

Gazzaniga *et al.* suggest the possibility that the initially produced single word response comes from the right hemisphere which may be confabulated on by the left hemisphere which has not seen the picture but has heard the initial response of the right hemisphere.

Reports are only just emerging on the patient V.P., a 27-year-old right-handed female who underwent the two-stage commissurotomy in April 1979. Seizures began at 6 years. V.P., like P.S., seems on testing to have a bilateral representation for language, although the left hemisphere is superior, and she too is developing a right hemisphere capability for expressive speech (Sidtis, Volpe, Wilson, Rayport, and Gazzaniga, 1981).

> At our first evaluation (4 months post operative), she could not name any stimuli presented to her left sensory field. By the 12th post operative month, however, she named 32% of the left visual field words presented in one test. After such naming occurred, she often expressed surprise at these responses and demonstrated no insight as to why they were emitted (Sidtis *et al.*, 1981, p. 330, Note 4).

For V.P., Gazzaniga, Smylie, Baynes, Hirst, and McCleary (1984) showed that her right hemisphere was as good as her left hemisphere at naming written nouns and verbs of varying frequency. When the hemispheres were independently shown more complex scenes, however, interesting qualitative differences were shown between the responses of the two hemispheres. When the left hemisphere was shown a picture of an athlete jumping a hurdle it gave the following response:

> I don't know if he's an athlete or not, but he is a man running over hurdles. He's got gym shorts on, and I don't know for sure if he had a shirt on. I think he did . . . and tennis shoes, jogger's shoes.

The right hemisphere response was as follows:

> An athlete . . . a basketball guy? . . . had a uniform. His back was facing me, and he was on an angle. He looked like he had been walking, and he was gonna take another step because one foot was like more out.

So both hemispheres could describe the main features of the picture. As with P.S., the right hemisphere pictures were invariably characterized accurately, but then embellished. While the original description is probably the right hemisphere, the later embellishments appear to be the result of the left hemisphere hearing this description and adding its own guesses as to what is depicted in the picture.

Studies with P.S. have led the investigators to propose 'some covert neural mechanism' (Gazzaniga *et al.*, 1982, p. 61) that transfers phonetically or articulatorily based information from one hemisphere to the other in this individual. They conclude from their series of experiments that information is not transferred via simple sensory means or overt cross-cueing, or via the intact anterior commissure, but phonetically rather than semantically via some other paracallosal route. A reasonable guess by the group is that P.S. has bilateral representation for speech production, which takes over from independently generated hemispheric processing at the level where the phonetic specification is translated into articulatory commands. This interesting observation suggests that the point of divergence from independant lateral control to bilateral control is where a more abstract specification becomes a more concrete neuromuscular programme. Anatomically, this might be at the level of the basal ganglia, although Gazzaniga's group point out that paracallosal transfer could take place at more than one level available to both right and left speech generation systems.

The developing linguistic abilities in the right hemispheres of these two patients, particularly the developing speech capability, have particular significance for the notions of plasticity and the function of the right hemisphere following unilateral left hemisphere damage. The evidence appears to demonstrate clearly that both patients have bilateral representation for language, but even so, as Gazzaniga *et al.* (1979, p. 813) point out with regard to P.S.:

> acknowledging the early left temporal seizures of this unusual man does not help to explain the progressive development of speech in the right hemisphere.

A number of explanations seem worthy of consideration. Firstly, P.S. cannot be dismissed as a freek occurrence as there are now two patients who appear to have a right hemisphere capable of developing language and speech. Both have long histories of epilepsy and had significant bilateral representation for language pre-operatively, but then there were patients in the Bogen–Vogel series who had bilateral representation also, so this can be no more than a contributing factor. It may be that the surgical procedure itself has contributed. The current Wilson procedure employed for P.S. and V.P. entails two phases where the initial phase involves section of the anterior portion of the corpus callosum (but not the anterior commissure) followed by a second operation some seven weeks later to complete the sectioning of the corpus callosum (Wilson, Reeves, and Gazzaniga, 1978). It is at least conceivable that the first phase may have caused some hemispheric reorganization. Finally, both patients appear to be undergoing intensive study, being tested at monthly intervals at least. Whether this is more intensive than investigations on earlier split-brain patients is not clear, but it just may be the case that such relatively intensive right hemisphere stimulation in patients who already have bilateral representation for language could encourage the development of a speech production capability in the right hemisphere. If this is indeed the case, then this would support an approach to treatment of aphasia which aimed to encourage new learning in the right hemisphere using lateralizing techniques. We return to this point in Chapter 8.

The split-brain evidence, therefore, indicates that the right hemisphere can develop speech production capabilities following separation from the left hemisphere in some neurophysiological circumstances in combination with some bilateral representation for language resulting from early brain damage. See Gazzaniga (1983) and Zaidel (1983) for recent lively argument. Next we examine those few useful reports of speech from mature individuals with only a right hemisphere.

SPEECH FROM THE ISOLATED RIGHT HEMISPHERE

In examining these left hemispherectomy and hemidecortication cases we bear in mind that most have not been well reported. There are very few mature cases and most were very ill people who did not survive for very long; but they show that speech can be produced in the absence of a left cortical hemisphere. Zollinger's (1935) female patient (A.C.) underwent surgery which left the medial part of the thalamus and a small portion of the globus pallidus. A.C. was able to respond 'all right' to all questions several hours after surgery, although it is not reported whether this was a perseverative or stereotyped response of some kind. The patient was able to say 'yes' and 'no' the day dollowing surgery and 'thank you' and 'sleep' on the second post-operative day. 'Goodbye' and 'please' were added on the next day, and Zollinger reports that on this day she 'showed a more accurate use of words' (p. 1060), implying that the patient's use of words up until the third post-operative day was to some extent inappropriate. Zollinger reports that some of the elementary vocabulary was actually taught by nursing staff and that he felt that vocabulary would have improved had the patient survived for more than 17 days.

Crockett and Estridge's (1951) male patient (G.S.) had surgery which spared half the globus pallidus, a third of the caudate nucleus, and all of the thalamus. Some hours after surgery G.S. was able to say 'yes' and 'no', and two weeks later 'No, I don't want any', and 'Put me back to bed'. Speech apparently improved and a few more simple words emerged until about one month after surgery when a 'block' of some kind occurred in his speech and he began to utter the apparently meaningless 'caw' and 'aw-caw'. Subsequent investigation at autopsy revealed a recurrence of the tumour involving the left surface of the pons in the midbrain and the basic pendunculi. From then on the patient's only utterances were 'aw-caw' and 'yes' and 'no' until his death four months post-surgery. There is no indication as to whether 'yes' and 'no' were appropriately used.

Hillier's (1954) younger patient, a 15-year-old Cherokee Indian boy, underwent left hemidecortication 'sparing as much of the basal ganglia as possible' (p. 720) and survived for 27 months. Sixteen days after surgery he was able to say 'mother', 'father', 'nurse', and 'similar expressions'. At discharge (30 days post-surgery), apart from apparently normal auditory verbal comprehension, Hillier reports that

the patient's vocabulary showed daily improvement though he had a tendency at first to respond to questions with 'I don't know'; persistent questioning, however, resulted in appropriate responses. He was able to call his physician and nurses by their names. He was possibly slightly euphoric (p. 720).

Before his death the patient is described as having a constantly improving 'motor' aphasia and anomia. Hillier concludes that 'there is evidence to suggest a strong transference of the left hemispheral functions to the remaining right cerebral hemisphere' (p. 721).

Smith's patient E.C. (Smith, 1966; Smith and Burkland, 1966; Zangwill, 1967) underwent a complete left hemispherectomy and a fuller examination. Smith reports that:

E.C.'s attempts to reply to questions immediately after operation were totally unsuccessful. He would open his mouth and utter isolated words, and after apparently struggling to organize words for meaningful speech, recognized his inability and would utter expletive or short emotional phrases (e.g., 'Goddamit'). Expletives and curses were well articulated and clearly understandable. However, he could not repeat single words on command or communicate in 'propositional' speech until 10 weeks post-operatively when he replied to a nurse (asking if he had had a B.M.), 'What does B.M. mean?'. Although E.C. is unable to speak voluntarily most of the time, occasional propositional speech continues to increase, along with ability to repeat successfully longer sentences on command in fewer trials (Smith, 1966, p. 468).

Propositional speech was reported to be limited, although present, and six months post-surgery E.C. was able to respond 'What do you think I am? A mind reader?' to the question, 'Is it snowing outside?', as well as other sentences and the words of several old familiar songs.

Zangwill's (1967) examination of E.C. at 18 months post-operation showed that the patient used 'yes', 'no', 'I don't know' always appropriately, as well as 'emotional' speech and expletives like 'No, God damn it, that's . . .', 'Yes, but I cannot . . .', 'God damn it yes' and 'Oh, my God'. He was able to repeat some words and name some objects and colours, while producing semantic paraphasias (he called a 'pencil' a 'pen' and the colour 'red' he called 'black'). He could count up to 20, but made errors. Zangwill states:

The impression made upon me by this patient was very much like that of a case of severe motor aphasia and right hemiplegia from left-sided cerebro-vascular accident (p. 1017).

The strong similarity between this patient's symptoms and severe Broca's aphasia leads Zangwill to continue:

82

this case has convinced me that, in this particular patient at least, the right hemisphere—possibly in association with subcortical mechanisms—was sustaining a measure of language (p. 1018).

What is of particular interest is that E.C.'s speech was more than non-propositional. A great deal of the patient's speech:

must be regarded as transcending emotional utterances and as essentially propositional (p. 1018).

These few reports show that the isolated right hemisphere is capable of speech production. It is only in E.C., however, that this speech is clearly seen to be propositional and where surgery was sufficiently radical to remove most left hemisphere subcortical structures. In addition, there are indications from E.C. and Hillier's patient that speech production improves with time post-surgery. Whether this apparent improvement represents developing right hemisphere capabilites or simply reflects a general improvement in health is not clear.

Language can also be expressed through writing. Before we conclude this chapter we look at those few studies which have sought to characterize the right hemisphere's contribution to writing.

WRITING

Little is known about the cerebral control of writing and few studies have addressed the question of the role of the right hemisphere. The evidence we have comes from a handful of sources, mainly where examination has been made of the written output of unilaterally right-hemisphere damaged patients (Kinsbourne and Warrington, 1962; Hécaen and Marcie, 1974; Simernits-kaya, 1974; Lebrun and Lebrun, 1971; Lebrun and Rubio, 1972; Lebrun, 1983). Patients with right hemisphere damage tend to reduplicate or omit strokes and letters, with reduplication dominating. Reduplication occurs also on numbers. Figure 2 shows this reduplication and deletion of strokes (notice also that the reduplication occurs especially on the letter 'm'). Errors can occur in direct copying as well as during spontaneous or dictated writing but are less prevalent in non-cursive, upper-case writing. In addition patients are unable to correct either their own or someone else's errors when they read over a text.

Lebrun (Lebrun and Lebrun, 1971; Lebrun and Rubio, 1972; Lebrun, 1983) has suggested that the errors in writing mode by right-hemisphere-damaged individuals occur as a result of impaired visual and kinaesthetic control and has termed the disorder 'afferent dysgraphia'.

The patient knows how the word should be spelled, but he is no longer able to ascertain whether he is implementing this spelling correctly in his writing, especially when the words contain sequences of similar strokes or curves (Lebrun, 1983, p. 31).

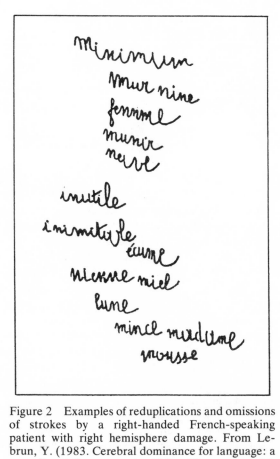

Figure 2 Examples of reduplications and omissions of strokes by a right-handed French-speaking patient with right hemisphere damage. From Lebrun, Y. (1983. Cerebral dominance for language: a neurolinguistic approach. *Folia Phoneatrica*, **35**, 13–39. *Reproduced by permission of S. Karger AG, Basel.*

Afferent dysgraphia, Lebrun suggests, is part of the more general disturbance in the processing of incoming spatial information, which fits well with the general notion of the right hemisphere's specialization for visuospatial processing.

Other features of right hemisphere dysgraphia can also be seen in Figure 2 which are explainable in terms of visuospatial impairment. There is a lack of horizontal placement of lines on the page and patients often write words over one another. If there is left visual neglect, the patient will use only the right side of the paper.

Hécaen and Marcie (1974) also characterized the disorder in terms of a visuospatial deficit when they described it as 'spatial dysgraphia'. They describe the same major features of the disorder as: reduplication of strokes, sometimes letters (particularly m,n,u) and very rarely syllables or words; lack of horizontal placement with lines slanting to either top or bottom of the page (some left-hemisphere-damaged patients, on the other hand, may fail to fill the right-hand side of the page); a tendency to leave spaces between graphemes within a word, sometimes placing separate graphemes on separate lines. Hécaen and Marcie report that the disorder occurred in 32 of 146 cases (21.9%) of unilateral right hemisphere damage, and that it can be significantly correlated with 'spatial dyslexia', accalcalia, left homonymous hemianopia, constructional apraxia, and unilateral spatial neglect. In a comparison of 52 right-hemisphere-damaged, 30 left-hemisphere-damaged, and 25 normal subjects on various writing tasks they found that right occipital lobe lesions were mainly associated with the disorder, but that horizontal orientation impairment appears to occur with left or right hemisphere lesions (although probably Rolandic and parietal lesions predominate in left-hemisphere-damaged patients). Although writing is often impaired following right hemisphere damage, most authors have explained the deficit in terms of an impairment of visuospatial processing which is intimately related to left unilateral neglect and other visuospatial and perceptual disorders. It has therefore been characterized as a non-linguistic disorder of writing.

However, Marcie (1983) has suggested that those explanations which propose a fundamental perceptual deficit ignore such 'linguistic' features of the disorder as the tendency to re-read the written material as if it were correct and did not contain errors as well as the finding that when right-hemisphere-damaged patients omit words when writing, they are often grammatical words. Levy, Nebes, and Sperry (1971) examined right hemisphere mediation of writing in the split-brain subject L.B. L.B.'s left hand was able to arrange two or three plastic letters screened from view into words (e.g., if, boy, can) on six out of six trials, although he was unable to say the words he had arranged. In an additional test L.B.'s left hand was presented with 10 high frequency two- to four-letter words (e.g., so, pet, soon) screened from view. Although he was unable to say the haptically presented word he was able to write correctly 9 out of 10 words. These findings indicate some linguistic mediation of some aspects of writing in the separated right hemisphere of this subject.

Simernitskaya (1974), however, has suggested that the differences between right and left hemisphere dysgraphia can be characterized in terms of the automatic–propositional dichotomy. Right hemisphere damage, he suggests, mainly affects automatic writing, while complex, voluntary, segmental writing is relatively preserved. This is reflected in the majority of errors occurring on vowels, which he considers to be realized more automatically; the major problem being a confusion between vowels which are similar. Simernitskaya (1974, p. 343) states that following a right hemisphere lesion:

> the process of complex coding can be preserved while the immediate, automatic processes can be severely disturbed. That is why in these processes the restitution of the damaged function can be provided by a shift of the process towards

the higher, conscious level of organization and by a step-by-step analysis of the components involved in action.

This attempt to explain right hemisphere dysgraphia as a breakdown in non-propositional–automatic functions is interesting, but automatic aspects of writing are, *a priori*, those which will be affected by neglect and attentional problems. Horizontal orientation, omission, and reduplication errors would also appear to be more parsimoniously explained in terms of non-linguistic visuospatial and attentional impairment, although an impairment of automatic processing could account for these features also.

CONCLUSIONS

It may be useful to start the final section of this chapter with some reasonably firm conclusions.

1. The right hemisphere is not 'mute'.
2. The evidence from pathological automatic utterances in epilepsy, aphasia and other disorders, and that from hemispherectomy/hemidecortication studies, suggests that the right hemisphere may be involved in the processing of automatic–non-propositional speech.
3. There are indications from commissurotomy and mature left hemispherectomy studies that the right hemisphere is capable of processing propositional speech, perhaps only where there is some pre-existing bilateral representation for language and there has been unique neurophysiological interference with the brain.
4. The same source of evidence as in (3), and bearing in mind the same provisos, appears to imply that the mature right hemisphere may have the capacity to *develop* propositional speech production.
5. There is a little evidence from commissurotomy studies that the right hemisphere may mediate linguistically in some aspects of expression through writing.

It was the fundamental axiom of the dominance model that the right hemisphere was incapable of speech production. We have seen that evidence from a number of clinical sources using a range of investigatory procedures shows that this is not the case. We have spent some time in this chapter considering the propositionality dimension in language and its relationship to the hemispheres. Findings from a range of investigations with epileptic, hemispherectomy, aphasic, left-handed and other groups provide some support for Jackson's contention that the right hemisphere may be equally involved with the left in non-propositional–automatic–emotional speech production. Some evidence (i.e., rCBF) indicates that non-propositional speech processing may be more diffusely represented in the right than in the left hemisphere (Skinhoj and Lassen, 1980) providing some support for Semmes (1968) diffuse–focal model, while Wada studies suggest that speech production may be divided between the hemispheres along a propositionality dimension in some left-handers (Milner, 1974). Moreover, data from some individual commissurotomy and left hemispherectomy patients suggest that the right hemisphere is not only capable of propositional speech in certain unique circumstances, but may have the ability to increase propositional speech processing with time.

Despite some indications from split-brain studies that the right hemisphere may be involved in some linguistic components of writing, the findings from studies with the unilaterally right-hemisphere-damaged suggest that the right hemisphere's involvement appears to be limited to visuospatial processing alone. There is again here some suggestion that a history of epilepsy, some long-standing bilateral involvement in language, and drastic neurosurgical invasion of the brain may combine in such a way to enable more propositional features of writing to be mediated by the right hemisphere.

It is clear that comparisons between clinical groups, as well as comparisons between individuals within groups, show significant variability. There would appear to be both qualitative and quantitative differences between right hemisphere speech capabilities in different pathological groups. Thus, there is little evidence for right-hemisphere-mediated propositional speech in an intact but damaged brain, where the hemispheres are still capable of interaction. It seems that the nature and cause of the damage (e.g., commissurotomy, unilateral lesion, are apparently related to the amount and quality of speech that the right hemisphere can produce. (See Gazzaniga, 1983, and Zaidel, 1983, for discussion.) Overwhelmingly, the evidence for right hemisphere speech comes from clinical studies. There is little evidence, either positive or negative, which addresses the question of right-hemisphere speech in the normal brain. We should remind ourselves again, however, that this 'normal' right hemisphere belongs to a mature young (between 20 and 30 years), dominantly right-handed male. This constitutes only a subgroup of the population. A significant proportion of the human race is neither young, male nor dominantly right-handed. A not unreasonable interpretation of the pathological evidence that we have would be that the right hemisphere of a mature right-handed male may be involved in the processing of prosodic, emotional, and non-propositional features of speech production. Ultimately, the question of the role of the normal right hemisphere in speech production awaits the development of reliable and safe methods of investigation.

Chapter Five

THE ROLE OF THE RIGHT HEMISPHERE IN EXTRALINGUISTIC ASPECTS OF LANGUAGE

As stated earlier, there is more to human language than that which can be dealt with by a strictly linguistic (i.e., phonological, syntactic, lexical–semantic) model. In this chapter we examine the role of the right hemisphere in those aspects of language we shall dub *extralinguistic*. Extralinguistic is the generic term we shall employ to cover those important aspects of language not covered by a formal linguistic model. This will go some way towards overcoming a problem inherent in discussing such aspects of language, namely the terminological minefield characteristic of the area. A range of terms have been employed by different workers in this area with a glaring lack of inter-worker consistency. The literature is peppered by such terms as non-verbal, paralinguistic, pragmatic, prosodic, suprasegmental, and affective/emotional. Crystal (1969) notes that there are almost as many uses of the term 'paralinguistic', for instance, as there are writers on the subject. Some (Crystal, 1969) use the term as a category heading for vocal features which accompany speech (e.g., pitch, intonation), while others (Abercrombie, 1968) apply it to both vocal and non-vocal features. Others have used the term 'prosody', particularly in aphasiology and speech pathology (Monrad-Krohn, 1963; Darley, Aronson, and Brown, 1969, 1975; Kent and Rosenbek, 1982) to refer to such features as quality, intensity, and intonation.

Phonologists often use the term 'suprasegmental' to refer to some of these features because their domain of influence extends beyond a single segment. An intonation contour, for instance, runs through an utterance made up of a number of words (Hyman, 1975). In practice, however, it is often difficult to decide whether a particular feature is functioning segmentally or suprasegmentally, linguistically or non-linguistically (Cutler and Isard, 1980). For instance, some Indo-Chinese languages use tone linguistically (Thai, for example). A word can have a completely different meaning depending on whether it is uttered on a high or a low tone (Van Lancker and Fromkin, 1973; Hyman, 1975). The problem concerning the *linguistic* contribution of suprasegmental features also extends to non-tone languages like English, however. Clearly, the variations in an intonation contour which can change a statement into a question carry significant linguistic weight. In this chapter those extralinguistic features of speech, such as intonation, pitch, and voice quality, will be referred to as *prosody* and disordered prosody as dysprosody or aprosody following the general usage in the clinical literature.

Those extralinguistic aspects of communication which come under the label of *pragmatics* are also relevant to the issues discussed in this chapter. Pragmatics represents an interface between language and other aspects of behaviour and is concerned not with linguistic entities themselves but with the total behavioural–social context in which communication takes place, and the actual intentions behind an utterance or message. There has been an increased appreciation of the importance of pragmatics in recent years reflected in development in linguistics, psycholinguistics, sociolinguistics, and speech and language pathology. An important function of language is to communicate affective or emotional states and the right hemisphere has been heavily implicated in both the control of emotion and the processing of affective/emotional language. We examine in detail the links between emotional language and the right hemisphere, and for practical reasons, if for nothing else, subsume affective/emotional aspects of language under the catch-all of extralinguistics.

Recent research has examined hemispheric contributions to pragmatic, prosodic, and emotional aspects of communication, and in this chapter we examine the evidence for a special role for the right hemisphere in the processing of the extralinguistic aspect of communication. Such a notion, that one hemisphere is responsible for linguistic and the other for extralinguistic forms of communication, is a neat and very attractive idea, and of considerable theoretical interest. We examine first the evidence which has implicated the right hemisphere in pragmatic behaviour. We then look at investigations into prosody and emotional communication in separate sections.

PRAGMATICS

Most of what we know about the involvement of the right hemisphere in pragmatic aspects of language comes from the pioneering series of studies completed by Gardner and his associates with unilaterally right-hemisphere-damaged patients. Here we will look at the results of this series of studies (reviewed recently by Wapner, Hamby, and Gardner, 1981, and by Gardner, Brownell, Wapner, and Michelow, 1983) in some detail. The pragmatic abilities examined most closely by the group have been narrative processing and sequencing and linguistic–pragmatic appreciation of humour.

A range of tasks have been used by Gardner and colleagues to examine these complex linguistic abilities in the right-hemisphere-damaged. The battery of tests included one which was composed of four stories with different contents, each authored in such a way that additional spatial, emotional or bizarre, non-canonical elements could be inserted. As well as this, a story recall and interpretation test was used where narrative processing was examined using a whole range of measurements.* The ability to arrange sentences was examined in the right-hemisphere-damaged where the subject was required to arrange in appropriate narrative sequence a set of seven written sentences where each set described either a temporal, spatial or categorical narrative sequence. Linguistically mediated humour appreciation was investigated by having subjects rate how funny they considered a variety of tape-recorded jokes and joke-like stories which varied in how funny they actually were. Other variables were whether the jokes were puns or puzzles, for instance, and whether subjects were deceived by the superficial 'trappings' of jokes (like unusual person or place names).

Subjects were classified on the basis of CT scan evidence into anterior, central, extensive, and posterior subgroups. Three control groups were also administered the test battery in most cases: normal adults less than 65 years old; a right-handed aphasic group less than 65 years old with unilateral left hemisphere damage due to CVA, with either anterior–non-fluent, posterior (temporo-parietal)–fluent and posterior–anomic aphasias verified by CT scans; a group of normal ageing controls (65 to 85 years) with negative histories of neurological disorder.

Results of this series of investigations firstly confirmed that right-hemisphere-damaged patients show no obvious signs of phonological or syntactic impairment, although the subjects showed a lack of ability to paraphrase material, often repeating whole elements of prose as in the original versions of the stories. The right hemisphere patients' performance on story recall showed that interpretation of spatial elements did not present too many problems, although interpretation of emotional and bizarre elements presented certain difficulties. For instance, failures in identifying the correct emotional feelings of characters in the stories were often confabulated and elaborated upon in a logical manner:

> Though often at varience with the emotions implied in the stories, the emotions stated by the patients were typically ones that could logically have been involved. Characteristically, the patients made inferences about how a character *could* have felt but not how he/she actually felt (Gardner *et al.*, 1983, p. 178).

Errors in interpretation of bizarre elements were the most marked for the right-hemisphere-damaged group. Unlike most of the control subjects, they tended to accept such elements and even added explanations to justify them:

> For example, asked why, in one story, a lazy hired hand had received a raise, patients were quick to justify the sentence. Four typical responses were: 'The

---

* The measures included scoring subjects on overall output of correctly or incorrectly assigned character traits and actions; noting confusions where incorrectly assigned character traits and actions were produced; scoring the subjects' ability to recall the six main events of the story; measuring the number of confabulations produced; noting the number of errors the subjects made in sequencing the events in a story; assessing the subjects' ability to produce an accurate version of the moral of the story.

cost of living is up'; 'Maybe he thought he wasn't paying him enough'; '... to encourage him to work a little harder'; 'He thought he was such a good worker he'd give him a raise' (Gardner *et al.*, 1983, p. 179).

Although ageing controls made errors in recall of elements and embellishment of the stories these errors were reported to be predominantly characterized by word-finding difficulty and personal remarks of a moralistic nature.

On the story recall test involving recall and interpretation of a fable-like story (The Silver Hammer), right-hemisphere-damaged patients did relatively worse with respect to overall output and recall of main story events than all controls, except the left-hemisphere-damaged aphasic patients. Right hemisphere patients made the most sequencing errors and produced the most confused story renderings, and together with the ageing subjects, the most confabulations. Right hemisphere patients also had marked problems in extracting the correct moral from the story, as did the ageing and aphasic groups.

Right-hemisphere-damaged patients had marked problems in organizing sentences into coherent narratives on the sentence arrangement test, as compared to normal controls. In fact, their performance was not much better than the aphasic groups. In addition, the poor performance of the right hemisphere group was not due to particular problems with temporal, spatial or categorical items, but seemed to reflect a definite impairment in organizing linguistic information at the narrative level in the absence of basic linguistic processing problems.

Humour appreciation was the other major area examined in right-hemisphere-damaged patients by the group. Results here showed that although right hemisphere subjects responded similarly to normal subjects on truly humorous material, they tended to react to non-humorous material as if it too were funny. Both groups rated the funniness of such items as puns, puzzles, and tricks similarly across items but rated the funniness within-types inconsistently compared to the ratings of normal subjects. Thus:

> the right hemisphere patients were able to appreciate some linguistically defined variation in humour (i.e., that puns as a kind of linguistic unit or class are funnier than are foils) but were unable to appreciate variations in funniness within type (Gardner *et al.*, 1983, p. 184).

When the funniness ratings of the separate subgroups of right hemisphere patients were examined it became clear that anteriorly damaged patients ($N = 2$) showed an 'elevated' or extreme humour response as compared to the other right hemisphere subgroups. This may have been due to the euphoria and anosognosia often present in such patients. In contrast the patients with posterior damage ($N = 2$) gave very low ratings suggesting an abnormally flat response to humorous material, possibly related to an association between posterior damage and depressed affect.

Overall, the results of these studies tend to indicate that right-hemisphere-damaged patients have problems with complex linguistic materials. They show a tendency to embellish and confabulate with a lack of sensitivity to the bizarre and emotional elements in narrative material. It may be, as the authors conjecture, that right hemisphere patients base their judgement on the plausibility of an element on the element itself rather than on the narrative context. It seems as if such patients have:

> problems in acquiring a sense of the overall gestalt or form of linguistic entities. Patients seem unable to appreciate the relations among the key points of a story or joke. The basic schema—the major episodes organized in a hierarchically appropriate manner—seems disturbed, if not totally destroyed . . . their inability to negotiate noncanonical elements, their frequent confabulations, embellishments, and injections of personal details, all suggest that the basic scaffolding of the story has not been apprehended (Wapner *et al.*, 1981, p. 30).

A tentative model which helps summarize the findings from these studies has been proposed by the group which characterizes the current position with regard to left hemisphere and right hemisphere contributions to linguistic and pragmatic behaviour (Wapner, *et al.*, 1981). A schematic representation, based on Wapner *et al.*'s conclusions, is attempted in Figure 3. At one end of the horizontal axis are certain 'straight' (Wapner *et al.*'s quotation marks) linguistic levels—phonology, syntax, and literal lexical entities—which require computational capacities. The other end shows more complex linguistic entities which entail non-literal information, jokes, stories, and metaphors. At one end of the vertical axis are context-free linguistic entities such as

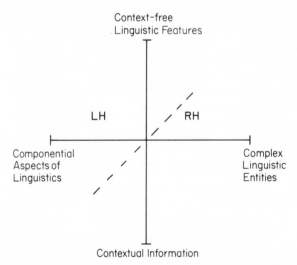

Figure 3   A graphic version of the model proposed by Wapner, Hamby, and Gardner (1981) of the hemispheric representation of linguistic and pragmatic processes. See text for explanation.

whether a sentence is syntactically correct or a story has an appropriate ending. At the other end are situations where contextual (pragmatic) information is casual, such as telling a joke, understanding the underlying intention of an utterance, and assessing the plausibility of facts within a story.

From the schematic representation of Wapner *et al.*'s conceptualization, it can be seen that complex linguistic entities which are dependent upon contextual information (pragmatic aspects) are the responsibility of the right hemisphere, componential aspects of linguistics which are not dependent on contextual features are subserved by the left hemisphere.

PROSODY

If we require evidence for the interaction and interdependence of cognitive functions then we can do worse than turn to the complex interplay which appears to exist between prosodic features of speech and music. We spend a little time in this section examining recent research into the hemispheric processing of music and musical elements before extending our investigations into prosody.

Music and the right hemisphere

The hemispheric processing of music was cited by Bradshaw and Nettleton (1981), as an illustration of complementary specialization and as support for the analytic–Gestalt characterization of hemispheric function. The view which has been held since the early clinical studies of the 1950s that the right hemisphere is 'dominant for music' has been displaced by a more sophisticated and complex characterization. Gardner (1982), taking a bottom-up and top-down approach, has intimated that while certain bottom-up elements which make up a musical piece may be processed by the left hemisphere, the actual top-down, holistically organized musical piece may be processed by the right hemisphere. While there is some support for this position, and such a hypothesis cannot be rejected on evidence currently available, the results of recent studies suggest that the hemispheric processing of music depends on a complex interaction of individual and task hemisphericity, individual levels of musical skill, degree of familiarity with the musical material, and experimental task requirements. There are also indications that while individuals who are not trained or skilled musicians depend on right hemisphere processing for music, trained musicians employ a fundamentally left hemisphere system. In a dichotic study, Bever and Chiarello (1974) found a right ear advantage in trained musicians and a left ear advantage in non-musicians in a melody recognition task. They suggested that the musicians employed a trained analytic approach, whereas the non-musicians used a holistic one which was not concerned with the separate componential elements of the melodies. Gordon (1975) produced similar results and conclusions for melody recognition and also (Gordon, 1978) for musical chords, as did Johnson (1977) using the recognition of violin melodies. Also using dichotic listening, Johnson, Bowers, Gamble, Lyons, Presbury, and Vetter (1977) found that trained musicians who were good transcribers as well as good readers, made fewer errors with melody identification at the right ear. However, when presented with a random note sequence they showed a left ear advantage. Less skilled musicians, unable to transcribe music, showed a left ear advantage for all types of musical stimuli.

Some EEG studies also support this general picture of more highly skilled musicians employing an analytic left hemisphere system and less skilled or untrained invididuals processing music using a holistic right hemisphere system. Davidson and Schwartz (1977) found that musicians showed no EEG differences while whistling the tune of a song or speaking the lyric. Untrained subjects, on the other hand, showed reduced alpha over the right hemisphere while whistling. In addition Hirshkowitz, Earle, and Paley (1978), also using EEG, produced evidence that non-musicians, but not skilled musicians, use right hemisphere processing during musical processing.

Related to the right hemisphere role in music is its apparent role in singing. Singing is of particular interest as it combines phono-articulatory activity and music. Whether, during singing, the production of lyrics or the musical framework is 'dominant' is mainly open to speculation, although the indications from the clinical literature are that the melody-producing component of singing helps to 'carry' the lyric-producing component. It is a common clinical observation that unilaterally left-hemisphere-damaged aphasic patients with very severe apraxia of speech show remarkably retained abilities to sing, especially over-familiar songs. Even patients who may have no other speech but a recurrent utterance can often produce acceptable snatches of well-articulated songs. There has been little systematic study into the singing abilities of brain damaged individuals. However, a recent study (Yamadori, Osumi, Masuhara, and Okobo, 1977) described the singing abilities of 24 Broca's aphasic patients. Of those, 21 (87.5%) were able to produce good melody and 12 (50%) were able to produce clearly the actual words of songs while singing. This was in spite of the very severe non-fluent character of their speech. For many Broca's patients the lyrics of songs can be articulated well during singing, but with great difficulty, if at all, in speech. At least one adult left hemispherectomy patient (Smith, 1966) was able at seven months post-surgery to sing lyrics with more facility than he was able to produce speech.

There are a number of cases in the literature of 'avocalia' (disorder of singing) consequent to right hemisphere damage cited by Lebrun (1983). He cautions that good reports have been few and handedness has not always been adequately described. The case described by Latham (1849) appears to have been the first to be reported. This patient received a blow to the right parietal area and the avocalia was apparently the only problem he suffered when consciousness was regained. From being very fond of singing and whistling the patient became unable to sing familiar songs or learn new ones.

We have seen that, for right-handed individuals, untrained in music at least, the right hemisphere appears to play the major role in processing aspects of music and the production of song. Whether the right hemisphere is responsible for the production of the lyrics of a song as well as the melodic carrier, is unclear, though the evidence from the clinical studies would suggest that this may be the case. As we have seen earlier (Chapter 1), many workers in this field have felt the need to characterize the contribution of the two hemispheres to the processing of different musical elements in terms of a left-analytical/segmental and a right-holistic/Gestalt dichotomy. Next we examine the evidence for right hemisphere mediation of prosody.

Prosody and the right hemisphere

In the introduction to this chapter we have already mentioned the problems involved in deciding whether particular prosodic features are acting linguistically or propositionally, or being employed to convey emotional force. We discuss emotional aspects of language in the next section, and it will be appreciated that it is inevitable, and indeed desirable, that overlap will occur between this and the following section.

It is now generally accepted that the right hemisphere is involved in the processing of prosody. The evidence for this comes mainly from investigations of dysprody subsequent to unilateral right hemisphere damage in the absence of similar prosodic disturbance following left hemisphere lesions. Additional support comes from some dichotic studies with normal subjects.

A number of dichotic studies have produced evidence for right hemisphere or bilateral involvement in processing tonal sequences (Schulhoff and Goodglass, 1969; Haggard and Parkinson, 1971; Blumstein and Cooper, 1974; Zurif, 1974) as well as tonal sequences differing in emotional quality, which will be discussed in the next section. Dichotic evidence is also available for a right hemisphere or bilateral involvement in pitch (Efron and Yund, 1974; Yund and Efron, 1975; Gregory, 1982). Gregory's study, for instance, found that 75% of 222 subjects demonstrated a left ear advantage for pitch. Schulhoff and Goodglass (1969) presented 20 pairs of two-note and 20 pairs of three-note tonal sequences to 10 right-handed male subjects and observed a non-significant left ear advantage. Blumstein and Cooper (1974) filtered out the speech from four short utterances (a declarative, a question, a conditional, and an imperative) to leave intact the basic intonation contour. Subjects were required to decide whether a binaurally presented foil matched one of a previously presented dichotic pair, decide which sentence type the dichotically presented contours represented (linguistic condition), and match dichotically presented contours to a visual analogue (non-linguistic condition). A left ear advantage was obtained for all three conditions which was non-significant in the linguistic condition. These results might be interpreted to suggest that the left hemisphere becomes more involved as a function of the linguistic requirements of the task. This is supported by the finding that a right ear advantage is observed where tone is used phonologically to distinguish and contrast individual words, as in tone languages like Chinese and Thai (Van Lancker and Fromkin, 1973). However, Blumstein and Cooper carried out an additional dichotic test where sets of CV syllables were intoned as questions and imperatives, etc. Subjects were required to match one of the competing sequences to a following binaural contour. A significant left ear advantage was obtained on this 'linguistic' task. Commenting on this finding, Zurif (1974) makes the point that:

> not every feature useful in language is processed by the language dominant hemisphere. Indeed, it seems as if the intonation contour is one linguistic property that is better processed in the nonlanguage, right hemisphere (p. 393).

Work with brain damaged individuals in recent years has resulted in a new theory of right hemisphere control of prosody (Ross, 1981, 1983) which we discuss in some detail here. Dordain, Degos, and Dordain (1971, cited by Ross and Mesulam, 1979) observed voice changes including changes in pitch, volume and tone, in 17 right-handed patients with right hemisphere damage. Ross and Mesulam (1979) describe two patients with right hemisphere damage, one of whom showed serious impairment in the affective quality of her speech. She was left with an asthenic, monotonous, and colourless voice quality, which was probably closely related to a disorder of affect (she was also anosognosic). Ross and Mesulam's second case (left-handed) had 'a peculiar nonaphasic speech problem' (p. 145). This patient also suffered a right hemisphere lesion which caused a flat, expressionless, monotonic voice quality, which, he claimed, was not related to his emotional state. He reported that he was unable to match the tone of his voice with his mood. Like the first patient, his ability to 'feel emotion' inwardly was not affected. There were indications, however, of an accompanying disorder of affect, but this was more apparent than real according to the authors, in so far as the patient's voice quality was giving a false impression of his inward emotional state. For both of these cases CT scans revealed posterior–frontal supra-Sylvian lesions, with some damage to the basal ganglia.

Ross (1981, 1983) has extended observations on the effects of right hemisphere damage on prosody to advance a theory of right hemisphere specialization for prosody which mirrors the classical left hemisphere model for language. His theory of the *aprosodias* predicts that different forms of aprosody will result from damage to different anatomical areas of the right hemisphere. Moreover, these aprosody types will be observed to be analogous to the aphasia types resulting from damage to homogeneous areas of the left hemisphere. Taking eight classical forms of aphasia (motor (Broca's), sensory (Wernicke's), global, conduction, transcortical motor, transcortical sensory, anomic mixed transcortical motor, and sensory), defined in terms of the presence versus absence of four behavioural characteristics (fluency/non-fluency, good versus poor repetition, good versus poor auditory comprehension, and reading comprehension), the theory predicts that eight forms of aprosody are possible (motor, sensory, global, conduction, transcortical motor, transcortical sensory, anomic, mixed transcortical motor and sensory). The aprosodias are defined in terms of the quality of prosodic abilities in four areas (spontaneous prosody and emotional gesturing, prosodic–affective repetition, prosodic–affective comprehension, comprehension of emotional gesturing). These prosodic impairments, Ross suggests, are direct analogies of the observable linguistic impairments of aphasia.

Ross (1981) describes 10 non-aphasic right-hemisphere-damaged patients (and reports that a further 8 (Ross, 1983) have also been observed) who all presented with aprosody. Moreover, in 8 of these patients CT scans revealed that areas of the right hemisphere were damaged producing aprosodias which were anatomically homologous to left hemisphere lesions causing analogous forms of aphasia (see Figure 4). Thus, three patients with motor aprosodia (analogous to Broca's aphasia) had anterior–parietal, supra-Sylvian lesions and the aprosodia was characterized by monotonous voice, impaired spontaneous gesturing, poor prosodic–affective repetition, but intact prosodic–affective comprehension and visual comprehension of emotional gesturing. In contrast, one patient was described with sensory aprosodia (equivolent to Wernicke's aphasia with left hemisphere damage) whose CT scan showed a right hemisphere posterior–superior temporal and inferior–posterior parietal lesion. This patient presented on examination with intact prosodic variation and spontaneous gesturing, but impaired prosodic–affective comprehension, prosodic–affective repetition, and visual comprehension of emotional gesturing. Other forms of aprosodia were described with CT scan evidence to support the theory. However, two patients who were described as having transcortical aprosodia had CT scan results which did not show lesion distribution in the right hemisphere analogous with the areas of damage to the left hemisphere producing transcortical motor aphasia. In addition, no aprosodic equivalents to anomic or conduction aphasia were described.

Some of the predictions of this characterization of prosodic impairment following right hemisphere damage have therefore been confirmed by Ross, but as Kertesz (1983) observes,

> this attractive proposal, almost too logical and simple to accept without reservations, undoubtedly will challenge others to verify it by careful quantification (p. 518).

Indeed, Lebrun (1983) has raised a number of questions concerning Ross's theory. He points out that two of the patients at least had dysarthria which could account for some of the impaired prosody and two of the motor 'aprosodics' had some history of anosognosia which may indicate that their flat monotonic and uninflected speech was a reflection of their indifferent attitude and concern. Lebrun also notes that an unambiguous aprosodic equivalent of paraphasia has not been described in right-hemisphere-damaged patients.

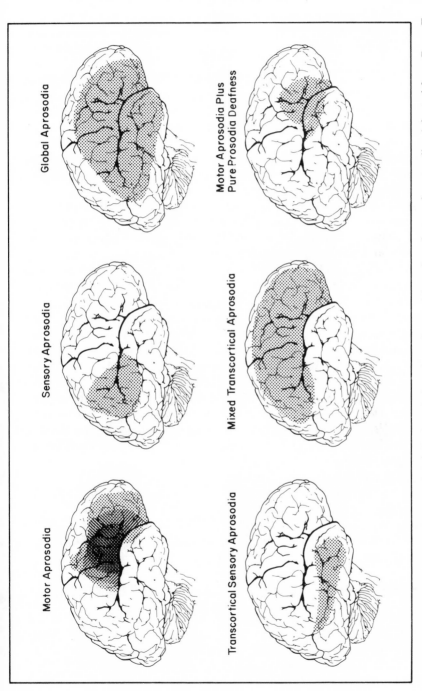

Figure 4 CT scan derived sites of right hemisphere lesions in patients with various forms of aprosodia. Adapted from Ross, E. (1981). The aprosodias: functional–anatomic organization of the affective components of language in the right hemisphere. *Archives of Neurology*, **38**, 561–569. Copyright 1981, American Medical Association.

Affective paraprosody, as Lebrun calls it, would be predicted to be a common result of posterior right hemisphere damage on Ross's model, where 'the occurrence of affective intonation patterns which do not fit the semantic contents of the sentences they are superimposed upon (Lebrum, 1983, p. 29) would be expected.

Ross's theory may seem somewhat premature given the amount and quality of evidence at present available. Clearly, support for the theory depends on future research concentrating on demonstrating double dissociation between the kinds of aprosody described by Ross following right hemisphere damage and the prosodic disturbances which accompany left hemisphere damage. Prosodic aspects of language are by no means as intact following left hemisphere damage as has been traditionally thought (Danly and Shapiro, 1982; Danly, Cooper and Shapiro, 1983; Foldi, Cicone and Gardner, 1983), although the indications from some acoustic studies are that the dysprosody of Broca's aphasia may be more closely related to linguistic (agrammatism) and phonetic (apraxia of speech) disruption than to a primary prosodic dysfunction (Danly and Shapiro, 1982; Foldi et al., 1983).

Shapiro and Danly (1985) have recently produced some acoustic evidence that right hemisphere damage can produce a prosodic deficit which is independent of affective disturbance, providing some support for Ross's model. They conducted an acoustic analysis of the performance of three patients with anterior, three with central, and five with posterior right hemisphere damage on tasks which involved reading aloud target sentences embedded in paragraphs, while intoning their voices in either declarative, interrogative, happy or sad modes. The performance of the right-hemisphere-damaged patients was compared with that of five posterior left-hemisphere-damaged patients, and five neurologically normal controls. When compared to the performance of the left-posterior patients (mildly aphasic) and normal subjects, the right-anterior and right-central patients spoke with reduced pitch variation and restricted intonation range while right-posterior patients produced exaggerated pitch variation and intonation range.

Future studies should aim to control more carefully for the effects of dysarthria, as prosodic disturbances are inevitable consequences of many dysarthria types (Darley, Aronson, and Brown, 1969, 1975; Kent and Rosenbek, 1982), and seek more objective instrumental verification and analysis (Danly and Shapiro, 1982; Kent and Rosenbek, 1982; Code and Ball, 1984). Kent and Rosenbek, for instance, carried out spectrographic analysis on the prosodic patterns of three mildly dysarthric patients with CT scan evidence of lesions limited to the right hemisphere. The most marked feature was a close similarity to the kinds of patterns produced by patients with Parkinson's disease, including normal or fast rate of utterance, reduced acoustic contrast, and diminished energy in the higher frequencies. This pattern produces flat, monotonic, indistinct, and hypernasal speech. This kind of pattern could easily give the impression of depressed effect, although there was no indication in the study that the patients had depressed effect.

Ultimately, the test of Ross's model and the whole hypothesis that the right hemisphere plays some special, maybe superior, maybe dominant role in the processing of prosody, depends on future studies which control for the presence of dysarthria and disordered affect, and manipulate these variables to allow subgroup comparisons.

In the final section of this chapter we extend our investigation into the emotional function of prosody when we examine the links between prosody and the right hemisphere's role in emotion.

EMOTIONAL LANGUAGE

Emotion and the right hemisphere

The notion that the right hemisphere has special involvement in emotional aspects of language goes back at least to Jackson, who suggested that:

> there are two modes of expression, one emotional and the other intellectual. By one we show what we feel, and by the other we tell what we think (1866, p. 121).

The right hemisphere, he considered, was concerned with the former and the left with the latter. Recent research in the area, especially the present surge of tachistoscopic studies into the processing of emotional facial expression, indicates increasing support for Jackson's view. It would appear, however, that a major obstacle to progress in this area is the existence of several separate models of the cerebral representation of emotion, based on a mixture of clinical and tachistoscopic experimental evidence (Code, 1986).

There is the anterior–posterior or left hemisphere dominance characterization which derives predominantly from observations on left-hemisphere-damaged patients. The two major syndromes described by this model are classic: a non-fluent aphasia resulting from anterior left hemisphere damage with agrammatism and relatively intact comrehension, accompanied by a negative, depressive affect often referred to as catastrophic reaction; a fluent aphasia following posterior left hemisphere damage with paraphasia and severe comprehension deficit, tending towards the abnormally positive. Such patients are often euphoric and oblivious to their true condition and this is often described as an anosognosic indifference or denial (Benson and Geschwind, 1975; Brown, 1975).

Experimental findings, especially from tachistoscopic studies of the processing of facial expression in normal subjects, have suggested separate characterizations of the contribution of the right hemisphere to emotion. The right hemisphere model suggests that the right hemisphere is responsible for the control of most emotional behaviour (Schwartz, Davidson, and Maer, 1975; Ley and Bryden, 1980; Dekosky, Heilman, Bowers, and Valenstein, 1980), whereas a left–right model proposes that the right hemisphere is responsible for control of negative emotion and the left for control of positive emotion

(Reuter-Lorenz and Davidson, 1981). Again, there is clinical evidence to support both characterizations of right hemisphere involvement (Gainotti, 1969, 1972; Wexler, 1980; Ley and Bryden, 1981; Tucker, 1981).

Support for the left–right model comes from clinical reports which suggest that unilateral left hemisphere damage tends to produce a depressive affect, sometimes with emotional lability and catastrophic reaction, which is seen as characteristic uninhibited right hemisphere behaviour (this includes such emotional reactions as crying, swearing, anxiety, and agression), but right hemisphere damage produces the opposite elated or euphoric affect, sometimes with anosognosia (Gainotti, 1972; Hécaen and Albert, 1978; Ley and Bryden, 1981). The right hemisphere condition has been described by Cicone, Wapner, and Gardner (1980) as:

> an indifference to or denial of physical problems, a forced joviality coupled with a tendency to indulge in 'gallows' and sexual humour, and a general tendency towards social and emotional inappropriateness (p. 145).

Gainotti (1969) examined 150 right-handed patients with right or left brain damage and found that the incidence of catastrophic reaction was 62% with left hemisphere lesions and just 10% with right hemisphere lesions. However, anosognosia was found to be present in 38% of patients with right hemisphere lesions and just 11% in left-hemisphere-damaged patients.

If we turn for a brief moment to the psychiatric literature, we find that, although left hemisphere overactivation and maybe corpus callosum dysfunction have been most implicated in schizophrenia, right hemisphere deficits have been suggested in research with subjects suffering from affective disorders (see Tucker, 1981, for comprehensive review). In addition, a number of studies have found that the conversion reactions of hysterical neurosis occur significantly more often on the left side (Galin, Diamond, and Braff, 1977; Ley and Bryden, 1979). Typically, in hysterical neurosis, a prominent symptom is the physical or sensory 'disorder' which has no apparent organic cause, and may serve some kind of symbolic or defensive function enabling avoidance of particular behaviour. Such symptoms as blindness, deafness, paralysis, and aphonia occur and Ley and Bryden point out that they appear predominantly on the left side at a ratio of 2 to 1. This, they propose, supports the emotional/affective right hemisphere hypothesis.

The confusing situation is not much improved when we turn for answers to more objective forms of evidence such as the results of sodium amytal studies. In a series of such studies reported by Rossi and Rosadini (1967), 73 subjects suffering from a range of neurological, or in some cases psychiatric, conditions were tested. Left-sided (left hemisphere) injection produced a depressive affect in 62% and euphoria in 38%, whereas right-sided injection produced depression in 16% and euphoria in 75%. Although these results would appear to support the left–right model, they suggest that it is not the case that the right hemisphere is responsible for positive and the left for negative emotional processing in all individuals. Moreover, Milner (1967) reports sodium amytal results which failed to replicate those of Rossi and Rosadini, and in fact produced a very different picture. Of 104 patients, 40 (39%) showed the same mood change with injection to either hemisphere—mostly euphoria. Of the others, 39 (37%) were more euphoric after left rather than right-sided injection and 25 (24%) were more euphoric following right-sided injection. Depressive reaction was seen in only 5 (4.8%) patients. The major discrepancies between these two sets of results can no doubt be accounted for in some measure by differences in size of barbiturate dose between the studies, perceptions of emotional state between experimenters, neurological and psychiatric state of the subjects, and even the well-known emotionally volatile nature of Italians when compared to Canadians!

Unfortunately there is no shortage of conflicting findings in this developing area or of results which are difficult to interpret in terms of the existing models. 'Differences' emerged in a recent study which compared the galvanic skin responses (GSR) of right-hemisphere-damaged and left-hemisphere-damaged subjects and controls while they were viewing emotionally loaded and neutral slides (Morrow, Vrtunski, Kim, and Boller, 1981). Right-hemisphere-damaged subjects produced virtually no GSRs to either emotional or neutral material, and left-hemisphere-damaged subjects showed decreased GSRs in comparison to the normal subjects.

Dimond and Farrington (1977) monitored heart rate while subjects were shown a film of a surgical operation. The film was shown either to right or to left hemisphere using a contact-lens method which allowed extended visual exposure. In another study (Dimond, Farrington, and Johnson, 1976) subjects rated how horrific they found the film. Results from these studies showed greater left hemisphere involvement in positive and right hemisphere involvement in negative affect. We discuss further the usefulness of the existing models later in this chapter. We turn now to the question of right hemisphere involvement in the language and communication of emotion, and begin with facial expression.

The communication of emotion via facial expression

We consider below the current work which is focusing on the nature of the right hemisphere's involvement in the communication of emotion via facial expression. The central importance of the face in human experiences is illustrated powerfully by the position it has enjoyed in all cultures since the dawn of art to the present (Gombritch, 1968). Faces seem special for human beings, and maybe the processing of facial information by the right hemisphere is special (for reviews see Benton, 1980; Young and Ratcliff, 1983; Rinn, 1984), and can be granted the unique kind of status in the right hemisphere that language enjoys in the left. Alternatively, rather than there being anything particularly unique about it, the processing of facial information may be a relatively unextraordinary reflection of the right hemisphere's general underlying visuospatial and Gestalt processing abilities (Bradshaw and

Nettleton, 1981). A further alternative emphasizes the interrelationships which appear to exist between emotion and facial recognition; a relationship where emotion is seen as the dominant and senior partner. Here, the facial *expression*, rather than the face *per se*, is what underlies the apparently superior right hemisphere involvement (Borod, Koff, and Caron, 1983a).

Most of the tachistoscopic work which has examined hemispheric processing of appreciation of facial emotional expression has supported the position that the right hemisphere is superior for the processing of emotion, whether negative or positive (Suberi and McKeever, 1977; Ley and Bryden, 1979; Dekosky, Heilman, Bowers, and Valenstein, 1980; Strauss and Moscovitch, 1981; Duda and Brown, 1984). Some of these studies, however, did show a non-significant right hemisphere superiority for certain negative emotions, and other studies have shown that the right hemisphere is superior in processing negative and the left is superior for processing positive emotional facial expression (Reuter-Lorenz and Davidson, 1981; Reuter-Lorenz, Givis, and Moscovitch, 1983). But Duda and Brown (1984) failed to replicate the reaction time results from Reuter-Lorenz and Davidson (1981). They found a clear right hemisphere superiority for positive emotional facial expressions presented tachistoscopically and no significant visual field differences for negative emotional expressions. They suggest that the database for the Reuter-Lorenz and Davidson study was rather limited. Natale, Gur, and Gur (1983) conducted a series of tachistoscopic experiments which examined the involvement of the hemispheres in processing emotional valence of facial expressions and provided support for differential involvement of the hemispheres in positive and negative emotion. Their Experiment I showed that right-handed subjects (but not left-handed subjects) rated emotional expressions as more negative when presented unilaterally to the left visual-field, suggesting a right hemisphere which is biased towards negative, but not positive, emotion. Experiment II presented happy, sad, and mixed chimeric faces to the visual fields. The two halves of the presented face expressed either the same (i.e., happy or sad) or opposite (i.e., happy and sad) emotions. Left visual-field presentations were judged more accurately, suggesting a right hemisphere superiority for judging emotional valence, probably at a fairly preliminary stage of information processing, as the fast exposure durations only allowed recognition of the presence of a face but no time to process the emotional expression.

Experiment III examined the possible bias of either hemisphere which may permit processing at higher stages of information processing. Mixed (happy and sad) chimeric faces were presented at exposure durations determined to allow recognition of the fact that the faces expressed two emotions, without allowing the subject to determine whether the expression was positive or negative. A left hemisphere bias to rate mixed faces as positive was obtained with no right hemisphere bias. This result was interpreted to suggest that the left hemisphere is biased towards perceiving emotional expressions as positive.

Moving on from research on appreciation or perception of emotional expressions, a number of studies have found asymmetries in actual production of facial expression in normal subjects (Campbell, 1978; Sackheim, Gur, and Saucy, 1978; Borod and Caron, 1980; for reviews see Borod and Koff, 1983, and Sackheim and Gur, 1983). The general finding of these recent studies is that there is a greater intensity of emotional expression on the left side of the face in right-handed individuals.

It is known that the lower two-thirds of the face is supplied by a contra-lateral corticobulbar tract which extends from the motor cortex in each hemi-sphere to the nucleus of the facial nerve on the opposite side (Rinn, 1984; Sackheim, Weiman, and Forman, 1984). Such findings have lent support to the view that the right hemisphere is superior in the production of emotional communication via facial expression. In line with findings from other areas of hemispheric asymmetries research, sex differences have been found in the lateralization of facial expressions. Alford and Alford (1981) asked 129 male and 126 female undergraduates to wink as naturally as possible with one and then the other eye, and to raise their right eyebrow and then their left eyebrow independently. In a further study (Alford, 1983) 70 female and 38 male subjects attempted winking, eyebrow raising, mouth corner raising, nose wrinkling and mouth corner lowering. In both studies males displayed significantly greater left-sided facility than females. Of interest is the fact that asymmetries emerged in these studies on upper face actions. Also of interest is the intriguing finding of Moscovitch and Olds (1982) that there exists a large and universal minority of individuals (between 5% and 10% of the population) who can wink with only one eye. In their study, a significant number of 'one-eyed winkers' could wink only with the left eye. It has been suggested that the asymmetries which have been observed have emerged during posed facial expression, and that when displacement of facial muscle is measured during more spontaneously evoked expressions, significant asym-metries do not emerge (Ekman, Hager, and Friesen, 1981). However, significantly greater left-sided facial expression has been reported in spon-taneous as well as posed facial expression (Moscovitch and Olds, 1982; Borod, Koff, and White, 1983b; Dobson, Beckwith, Tucker, and Bullard-Bates, 1984). There is evidence to suggest that the two forms of facial expression may be separately organized in the brain (Borod et al., 1983b). Posed facial expressions are, by definition, deliberate, intentional and voli-tional, whereas spontaneous expressions are involuntary reactions to emo-tionally stimulating situations. The neurological evidence suggests that posed facial expressions involve the cortical pyramidal system whereas spontaneous expressions involve the subcortical extrapyramidal system (Moscovitch and Olds, 1982; Borod et al., 1983b).

Moscovitch and Olds (1982) conducted observational field studies of naturally occurring spontaneous expressions and found that most unilateral expressions occurred on the left side. In an additional laboratory experiment, 34 mixed sex and handedness subjects were asked to relate sad, funny or frightening experiences while being videotaped. Results showed that for right-handers unilateral facial expressions during speech were significantly more prominent on the left side.

A finding of particular interest from this study was observations on hand gestures which accompanied a facial expression and hand gestures which did not accompany a facial expression. They found a significant advantage for right-hand gestures which did not accompany a facial expression. The authors suggest that:

> this result further supports the idea that hemispheric dominance during speech shifts away from the left hemisphere and towards the right hemisphere whenever a facial expression occurs. At other times, the greater activation reverts to the left, 'speaking' hemisphere and is reflected in the predominance of right-hand gestures (Moscovitch and Olds, 1982, p. 77).

Borod *et al*. (1983b) also analysed posed and spontaneous expressions in a group of 37 right-handed male and female subjects. Subjects were videotaped while they viewed positive and negative emotive slides, while they attempted to pose expressions appropriate to particular slides and while they posed on verbal instruction to 'look happy' or 'look sad', etc. Both types of emotional expression were significantly left-sided, with negative expressions being left-sided for all subjects and positive expressions left-sided for males only. Females produced a less lateralized pattern with positive facial expressions being less lateralized than negative ones. The results of these studies do not support the idea that there exist different patterns of brain organization for posed and spontaneous emotional facial expressions.

The consistent finding from the research in the area is that the right hemisphere is crucially concerned in the appreciation and production of emotional messages via facial expression. The results on production of facial expression make an interesting contrast to the finding that something like 78% of subjects produce greater *right*-sided mouth opening *during speech*, implicating left hemisphere neural control of articulation (Graves, Landis, and Goodglass, 1982; Graves, 1983). The foregoing review suggests a strong case for a right hemisphere which is specially concerned with the processing of emotion and the production and appreciation of emotion via facial expression. More direct evidence for a dynamic interaction between emotion and emotional language is examined next.

Emotional language

A few dichotic studies have produced findings which support an interaction between emotion and language in the right hemisphere. Haggard and Parkinson (1971) examined ear advantages for emotionally toned sentences expressing anger, happiness, boredom and distress, while King and Kimura (1971) tested ear advantages for such non-verbal vocalizations as laughing and coughing. Carmon and Nachshon's (1973) dichotic study investigated laughing, crying, and shrieking in 29 mixed-sex subjects. All these studies observed a left ear advantage for such emotional vocalizations. A specialized right hemisphere ability to combine perception of facial expression with language is suggested by electrical stimulation research (Fried, Matser, Ojemann, Wohms, and Fedio, 1982). Fried *et al*. examined nine patients undergoing right-sided intracranical operations for intractable epilepsy. All were determined to have left hemisphere specialization for language on Wada testing. On electrical stimulation of an extensive area of the right cortex, it was the posterior portion of the middle temporal gyrus which produced significant errors in verbal labelling of emotional faces in four patients. Interestingly, the electrical stimulation caused no change in emotional set, or in perception of faces *per se*, but in the ability to label verbally the expressions in the absence of aphasia.

Graves, Landis, and Goodglass (1981) examined the degree to which the right hemisphere involvement in emotion extends to emotional language. In a lexical decision task they presented abstract emotional (e.g., fear, kill, rape, nude) and abstract non-emotional (e.g., time, view, dual, pile) words which were matched for frequency to the visual fields of 12 male and 12 female right-handed subjects. Words were mixed with pronounceable non-words and presented bilaterally and horizontally via a tachistoscope, and subjects were required to operate levers to make their decisions. Male subjects produced a significant left visual-field effect for emotional words, but female subjects produced a more variable pattern. This study demonstrates that the right hemisphere, for males at least, appears to have a special capacity for leading emotional words, which is independent of concreteness and imageability (as the words used in the experiment were abstract). Schwartz, Davidson, and Maer (1975) recorded the lateral eye movements (LEMs) of normal subjects while they were answering emotionally charged and neutral questions. Significantly greater left eye movements were observed during emotional than neutral questions. Tucker, Roth, Arneson, and Buckingham (1977) in a replication used the same questions as Schwartz *et al*. as well as including a stressful and non-stressful condition. They found that both emotional content and stress produced significantly more leftward LEMs indicating increased right hemisphere activation while answering emotionally charged questions and while under emotional stress.

A series of studies with brain damaged subjects has demonstrated the need for an intact right hemisphere for the correct comprehension and expression of emotional language. Wechsler (1973) examined the effects of right hemisphere damage on the ability to recall neutral and emotionally charged stories. Story recall was poor in right-hemisphere-damaged patients, particularly if the story was emotionally charged. Heilman, Scholes, and Watson (1976) compared the abilities of right- and left-hemisphere-damaged subjects to comprehend the content of spoken sentences and the mood of the speaker. The right hemisphere group were shown to have a significant deficit in making judgements about emotional mood during this task. Similarly, Tucker, Watson, and Heilman (1976) demonstrated that emotional communication via tone of voice is impaired following right hemisphere damage. The two right-hemisphere-damaged patients examined by Ross and Mesulem)1979), and described in an earlier context, also had what was termed a disorder of 'emotional gesturing' which accompanied their dysprosody. The first case showed a lack of facial expression conveying inward emotional states and there was a paucity of limb and body movements. The patient recovered from the disorder in six months, but the second patient still had problems five years post-stroke. With this patient 'the face was quite mask-like, there was a paucity of emotive movements that normally accompany speech and fluxes in mood' (p. 146). The impression made by these patients was the total inability to express emotion through speech or other forms of expressive action even when feeling strong emotions. One patient had even lost the ability to laugh and cry. Buck and Duffy (1980) examined emotional expression via facial expression and gesture in left- and right-hemisphere-damaged, Parkinson's disease, and normal subjects. The subjects' reactions to a range of emotional slides were rated by four male and four female judges. Left-hemisphere-damaged aphasic patients were the most expressive, followed (very closely) by controls. The group with right hemisphere damage were rated as less expressive than the previous two groups and the Parkinson's patients as the least expressive of all. Cicone, Wapner, and Gardner (1980) examined the sensitivity of 18 left-hemisphere-damaged and 21 right-hemisphere-damaged patients to emotional facial expressions, drawings of emotional situations, and written descriptions of emotional situations. They found that although aphasic patients had difficulties with the linguistic descriptions, the right-hemisphere-damaged patients showed a general reduction in emotional sensitivity illustrated by their poor performance on all tests. Right-hemisphere-damaged patients resorted to confabulation in many instances, produced bizarre descriptions based on misinterpretation of stimuli, and appeared to be insensitive to the overall polarity of emotions, suggesting a loss of sensitivity to relations between emotions. Cicone *et al.* suggest that this might indicate that such patients are able to infer permissible emotions, but their inferences are actually inappropriate.

Emotions: models of confusion

The evidence from the diverse sources that we have examined in this section leaves little doubt that the right hemisphere is involved in emotion and, moreover, that it enjoys some special function where emotional processing is concerned. It also suggests quite forcefully that mechanisms exist in the right hemisphere which mediate between emotion and the expression and appreciation of emotion through non-verbal and verbal means. This emphasizes one of language's most powerful functions, as a link between the outside world and our most private inner selves. It appears, furthermore, that the expletive, the soft loving tone, the harsh angry tone, the emotional break in the voice, the wink and the smile do not require componential or sequential synthesis or analysis. Their impact is immediate and their meaning is fundamental. What the data do not make clear yet, however, is the qualitative nature of the right hemisphere's role and to what extent it shares emotional processing with its neighbour. Borod, Koff, and Caron (1983a, p. 83) suggest that:

> It may be that the right hemisphere is specialized for emotion in the same way that the left hemisphere is specialized for language, with expression or production related to more anterior brain structures, and with appreciation or comprehension related to more posterior structures.

Although the data that Ross (1981, 1983) has presented in support of his anterior–posterior model of right hemisphere prosody lend some support to Borod *et al.*'s characterization, the evidence is, as yet, slim. The failure of replication and the lack of unanimity in the research can be put down to some extent to the current meteoric development of the area. The existence of the three models which were outlined in the introduction to this section is illustrative of this. While each model can claim support from the evidence available, they make conflicting and confusing predictions regarding the effects of localized brain lesions on emotion (Code, 1986). An anterior left hemisphere lesion will produce depressive affect on the anterior–posterior and left–right models, and have no effect on the right hemisphere model. However, a posterior left hemisphere lesion will produce anosognosic indifference on the anterior–posterior model, depressive reaction on the left–right model, and have no effect on the right hemisphere model. Moreover, an anterior right hemisphere lesion will produce depressive affect on the anterior–posterior model, positive affect on the left–right model and positive and/or negative affect on the right hemisphere model. Lastly, a posterior right hemisphere lesion will result in depressive reaction on both the anterior–posterior and left–right models; but euphoria and/or depression on the right hemisphere model.

Some of these predictions are borne out by clinical, experimental or psychiatric findings. It has been suggested (Code, 1986) that the confusion may have much to do with our inadequate understanding of the nature of emotion and emotional valence and the range of affective states that brain damaged patients present with. There has been little systematic research into the question, but it may be possible to identify separate forms of abnormally negative and positive affect in different patients resulting from damage to different brain regions and having different underlying causes. For instance, a specific visual anosognosia has been described (Hécaen and Albert, 1978) which may be a secondary effect of left unilateral neglect following right hemisphere damage. Clinical evidence suggests a highly significant correlation between anosognosia and unilateral neglect (Critchley, 1953; Gainotti, personal communication), and unilateral neglect occurs overwhelmingly for the left half of space following right hemisphere damage (De Renzi, 1977; Hécaen and Albert, 1978; Heilman, Watson, Valenstein, and Damasio,

1983). In contrast, the anosognosia noted in some posterior left-hemisphere-damaged patients may be related more to comprehension loss than to perceptual impairment. To what extent then may anosognosia following right hemisphere damage be seen in terms of a more fundamentally perceptual, than emotional disturbance? But, Tucker's (1981) recent review of the brain's control of emotion questions the traditional cognitivist position that emotion is ultimately controlled by 'higher' cognitive processes. The opposite position is that different forms of emotional arousal determine the kind of cognitive processing which is selected for any given task, suggesting that an individual's general cognitive orientation may be altered by particular emotional states.

A further possible source of confusion concerns the psychological appropriateness of emotional states following brain damage. It is by no means certain that depressive or manic states are direct and primary results of the site of lesion. There is evidence to show that a significant proportion of the mood change observed in brain damaged patients can be accounted for in terms of psychologically appropriate reaction. This may be true for depression (Robinson and Benson, 1981) and anosognosia (Weinstein and Kahn, 1955). The notion of inhibition is often invoked to provide existing models with more explanatory substance. On the dominance model, the normal balance of intrahemispheric inhibition is said to be disturbed following left hemisphere damage, whereas the left–right model resorts to interhemispheric inhibition for explanation. On the left–right model, the emergence of the abnormally positive state following right hemisphere damage is due to release of the left hemisphere from right hemisphere inhibition and the depressive affect of the left-hemisphere-damaged patient is due to the release of the right hemisphere from left hemisphere control.

It has been argued elsewhere (Code, 1986) that the very complexity of the relationships which exist between behaviour, cognitive processes, and brain mechanisms mediate against the simple subductive models that we have supported by all-powerful notions like inhibition. Grouping together all abnormal affective states into a neat catastrophic reaction–anosognosia dichotomy may be the source of much of our confusion where the cerebral processing of emotion is concerned.

CONCLUSIONS

The data conspire to present a picture of a right hemisphere which has special responsibilities for processing many non-linguistic aspects of language and communication. However, the current state of the research does not allow too many firm conclusions regarding a more exact characterization of right hemisphere involvement. The evidence as it stands cannot fully resolve the question of whether some superordinate right hemisphere mode forms the foundation for pragmatic, prosodic and emotional aspects of language, although findings have most often been interpreted in terms of the holistic right hemisphere idea. Similarly, a number of studies have suggested that relatively independent and dedicated mechanisms may underlie some extralinguistic skills, while others have implicated such right hemisphere functions as visuospatial, musical, and emotional processing as primary.

Despite this lack of unanimity, models have been proposed which account for some aspects of the right hemisphere's involvement in extralinguistic features of language. However, as we have seen, the findings from many clinical sources have been confounded by lack of control for the influence of associated disorders like anosognosia and dysarthria, and research in the entire area is frustrated by a lack of even operational agreement on the nature of such things as emotion and prosody.

Chapter Six

THE ROLE OF THE RIGHT HEMISPHERE IN THE RECOVERY OF APHASIA: THE LATERAL SHIFT HYPOTHESIS

It is a common and general observation in neuropsychology that the initial consequences of brain damage are more severe than the eventual consequences. This phenomenon has generally been seen in terms of 'recovery' of function. It was stated in Chapter 1 that the concept of lateral dominance began to take a firm hold on neurology (and subsequently, neuropsychology) with the findings of Broca (1865), and it was probably with Broca that the notion of right hemisphere 'take over' of language functions was first considered (Bogen, 1969b; Brown, 1979). Broca was not alone in this view, however. Both Jackson (1874) and Gowers (1887) discuss the possibility of the involvement of the right hemisphere in recovery from aphasia. This seems a logical implication of the dominance model in fact: having decided that one hemisphere is responsible for practically all language functions, it is then necessary to account for recovery from aphasia following widespread damage to that hemisphere. Thus, 'the lateral shift hypothesis', in some form, has a history going back to the latter half of the nineteenth century.

In its simplest form the lateral or hemispheric shift hypothesis states that following left brain damage there is a shift to the undamaged right hemisphere for language processing. The notion, in fact, is not a unified or cohesive theory. It represents, more like, a loose collection of clinical anecdotes and speculations, as well as conceptualizations based to some extent on clinical observations and experimental findings. Some ideas suggest that the right hemisphere is maximally engaged and plays the major role in recovery, while others propose that it is involved to a more limited and/or qualified extent. Others suggest that the right hemisphere becomes involved in more or less direct proportion to the amount of damage sustained by the left hemisphere's language-processing system. Still others entail the powerful notion that the right hemisphere may be prevented from greater participation by some form of suppression or inhibition from the 'dominant' left hemisphere.

VARIANTS OF THE HYPOTHESIS

Brown (1979) asks the questions:

Does the right hemisphere account for the various degrees of insufficiency in aphasia or is the right hemisphere truly aphasic? Is the right-hemisphere effect a compensatory one, in which a mirror system either limited in capacity or differing in design 'takes over' for the damaged side, or are structures in the right hemisphere part of a unitary bilateral organization mediating language? (p. 137).

This variety of claims for right hemisphere involvement in aphasia can, therefore, be grouped into three broad variants which should be theoretically distinguished from each other. The *first* of these suggests that any restoration observed in language is accomplished via some kind of functional substitution or reorganization. Such a position suggests that right hemisphere modes of cognition play a larger, compensatory, role following left hemisphere damage, whether spontaneously or as a specific result of rehabilitation or retraining. This position might be considered a weak form of the hypothesis, since it does not necessarily claim that strict linguistic functions *per se* are involved. The *second* broad variant claims that the right hemisphere does more than simply compensate for destroyed linguistic abilities, or even that it is capable of subserving linguistic skills beyond what might be expected, given what is known about right hemisphere abilities in other populations. This strong version of the hypothesis suggests that the right hemisphere takes on the responsibilities of the left: there is a complete shift of control of language. Thus, the mature right hemisphere is capable of taking on new skills; those skills which underlie linguistic processing which have previously only been possessed by the linguistically specialized left hemisphere. The *third* broad position is that the natural, residual, and pre-existing communicative capacities of the right hemisphere are all that remain following significant left hemisphere damage. Consequently, certain observed behavioural characteristics or symptoms of aphasia represent, not the distorted products of an impaired left hemisphere system, but the limited and particular language skills of the right hemisphere.

That the right hemisphere is involved in language processing is not in dispute. From this position it is a small step to suggest that the right hemisphere is involved in the communicative behaviour of aphasic patients. However, it is one thing to say that some observed communicative behaviour in aphasic patients represents the spared pre-existing competence of the right hemisphere, and it is entirely a different thing to suggest that the right hemisphere is responsible for any actual *recovery* from aphasia. There is obviously a significant theoretical distinction between, on the one hand, the claim that right hemisphere processing is responsible for a common aphasic symptom like phonemic paraphasia or some compensatory strategy like using a visually based communication system, and, on the other hand, the claim that the right hemisphere takes on responsibility for the actual control of language processing *in toto*. The first position ties in with a complementary specialization model of the representation of language in the two halves of the brain and the second broad position assumes that the left hemisphere has a dominant, controlling role over language which it relinquishes to the right following damage. This latter position therefore presumes that central control of 'the language system' is within the capacity of the right hemisphere, but that under certain neurophysiological circumstances, the left is reluctant to allow right hemisphere control for some reason. An essential component of this position is that of left hemisphere inhibition of right hemisphere capacity. We shall return to the question of interhemispheric inhibition later. In the remainder of this chapter we will attempt to sort through the mass of evidence for the variety of claims which have been made for hemispheric shift in aphasia.

MECHANISMS OF RECOVERY

Not only is it the case that a number of broad variants of the lateral shift hypothesis can be identified, but these represent only part of the even wider range of theoretical mechanisms which have been proposed over the years to account for observed recovery from brain damage. This collection is something of an hotchpotch of neurophysiological and behavioural explanations for recovery of function. Not only is the evidence in support of many of them very weak, but it seems clear that some explanations are not conceptually distinguishable from others. In addition, rather than explanations of 'recovery' some are really explanations of 'sparing' of functions. Some of these notions include the possibility of the participation of the right hemisphere in recovery from aphasia and we sketch the main features of the most relevant below. These mechanisms have been comprehensively reviewed by Rosner (1970, 1974) and Lawrence and Stein (1978) where more detailed discussion can be found. Lawrence and Stein classify these theoretical mechanisms as physiological, structural or process explanations, and refer to the latter two as 'conceptual' theories.

Physiological explanations include *diaschisis*, a mechanism originally proposed by von Monokow (1914). Diaschisis describes a theoretical situation where tissue at some distance from the lesion is negatively influenced by the radiation or spread of abolition of excitability via association fibres within one hemisphere (associative diaschisis), via the corpus callosum to the other hemisphere (commissural diaschisis), or via cortico-spinal pathways (cortico-spinal diaschisis). Thus, abolition of excitability within one neurone group is transmitted to other neurone groups closely adjacent to and closely related with the focally damaged area. Areas of brain which have fibre connections to the distrupted focus of damage will be affected by a 'wave of diaschisis'. The effects of diaschisis, therefore, are seen by von Monokow as being different from, and in addition to, the effects of the primary shock.

Functional impairments observed in brain damaged individuals are therefore the result of a combination of the primary focal damage and the reduced excitability of other components of the system related to the damaged area. Observed recovery is then seen as the reduction in the effects of diaschisis with residual functional deficits being more directly attributable to the original structural lesion. As von Monokow notes:

Complete recovery from diaschisis requires a certain time, but even before the recovery is complete (ups and downs) the inevitable local functional defects caused by structural disorders will become visible within the overall functional disorder, and this indicates the so-called residual stage representing the balance between the local injury and the counteraction provoked by that injury (1969, p. 32).

Recovery from aphasia with time and the emergence of some characteristic aphasic symptoms may be accounted for by the effects of a diaschisic form of interhemispheric inhibition:

In the case of commissural diaschisis certain innervation pathways in the intact contralateral hemisphere are inhibited by loss of continuity of fibres in the corpus callosum and other commissural fibres in the white matter of the affected hemisphere. In other words, massive lesions of commissural fibres in the left hemisphere will impair a number of more complicated nervous processes (apraxia, aphasia, agnosia). This associative type of diaschisis will inhibit the nervous function in those cortical points of the affected hemispheres which are connected by fibres to the area of the focus (von Monokow, 1969, p. 34).

Three related structural notions are those of *redundancy*, *multiple centres*, and *equipotentiality*. Redundancy refers to where the compromise of part of a system is compensated for by the rest of the system which has previously not been fully occupied. In this way it is conceived that a system can suffer neuronal loss without functional loss. Redundancy may be a structural conceptualization of the physiological explanation of relatively ineffective synapses. The essence of the notion of multiple centres is that more than one governing 'centre' is involved in the control of a given function. Recovery is due to remaining centres compensating for lost ones. Some overlap would appear to exist between this notion and that of redundancy. Equipotentiality is a structural explanation for recovery mainly associated with Lashley (1929), although probably originating with Munk (1881), which sees the brain, not as a collection of localized centres, but as a holistically organized system. On this notion most functions have representation throughout the brain and involve 'mass action' of the brain. Recovery of a function is achieved through remaining brain compensating for focally damaged brain.

The idea that a function involves activity at different hierarchically organized *levels of representation*, which are ontogenetically and phylogenically determined, is a structural explanation which originated with Jackson (Taylor, 1958). The idea still constitutes the central framework of neurology. The lack of control over laughing and crying that some pseudobulbar palsy patients experience, for instance, is seen as being due to the failure of higher level control. The upper motor neurone lesion has effectively disconnected the higher from the lower levels and higher systems can no longer exert influence over lower more primitive systems. What we interpret as recovery is the emergence of more primitive and automatic behaviour released from higher level inhibition.

Process explanations include *functional substitution* and *plasticity*. Functional substitution describes a situation where another undamaged functional system or subsystem can take over from a damaged functional system either spontaneously or through retraining. Patients with alexia may be aided to 'read' through presentation of material via the tactile modality (e.g., letters can be formed out of sand-covered card for presentation to the fingertips of the patient) or patients with severe apraxia of speech may be guided to articulatory placement through the use of visual diagrams. In both examples, surviving functional systems are substituting for damaged ones. Luria (1963, 1970; Luria, Naydin, Tvetkova and Vinarskaya, 1969) is a prominant advocate of functional substitution as a process of recovery and as a basis for therapy. Finally, the concept of plasticity proposes that radical neural reorganization can take place in response to brain damage. Plasticity was discussed in some detail in Chapter 2. There is clear overlap between the notions of plasticity and equipotentiality.

This series of theoretical explanations have been organized in a variety of other ways (Rosner, 1974; Powell, 1981; Miller, 1984). Rosner, for instance, classifies them under Jackson's hierarchical representation, Munk's and Lashley's substitution (equipotentiality), von Monokov's diaschisis and Luria's 'retraining' (functional substitution). He also refers to explanations which emphasize re-establishment of function and those that suggest replacement of lost function (Rosner, 1970). As Powell (1981) has observed, on some of these notions, it is astonishing that there is any loss of function at all following brain damage! In fact, some of these processes clearly describe not so much 'recovery' as 'sparing' of function, as is illustrated in the next section.

Le Vere's alternative view of recovery

However attractive and innovative some of these explanations for recovery might be it must be recognized that supportive evidence for many of them is often lacking. Le Vere (1975, 1980) has proposed an alternative view: behavioural recovery following brain damage is best explained with reference to the evidence that recovery of function is accounted for by the continuing operation of spared tissue.

> Conceptualizations of behavioral recovery suggesting other vaguely specified characteristics, such as functional reorganization, should at least for the present, be avoided. The reason for doing so is not simply a concession to parsimony but rather a respect for empirical findings (Le Vere, 1975, p. 356).

He suggests that:

> operational recovery following damage is dependent on what survives and what continues to function in the normal manner. From this point of view, behavioural recovery following brain damage is simply the result of the normal

mechanisms supporting the recovered function never being destroyed (Le Vere, 1975, p. 351).

In a later paper (Le Vere, 1980) this theory is developed to suggest that the actually observed behavioural deficit is the result of the individual's attempts to shift control to undamaged neural systems by way of compensation. Le Vere is here distinguishing between the behavioural deficit—the direct result of compensation—and genuine recovery of lost function. Genuine recovery is achieved through utilization of whatever is spared of the neural system directly affected by the lesion. The term 'recovery of function', he suggests, should be reserved to refer to the reinstatement of the specific behaviour which was disrupted by the brain lesion.

A potentially important consequence of Le Vere's theory from the point of view of rehabilitation is that,

> disrupted behaviours are, or may be, temporary and ultimately recoverable, but losses, whether measured behaviourally or neurologically, are just that—losses . . . Not only is recovery of function dependent upon morphological sparing, but also, because we postulate that the nervous system is incapable of reorganization and vicariation, recovery of function is dependent upon functional sparing (Le Vere, 1980, p. 300).

A behavioural deficit can occur, of course, even when the critical neural mechanisms are spared. But this occurs because the individual does not utilize surviving capacity in the damaged sytem, but tries to compensate for the effects of the damage by using other undamaged neural systems. Here, the lost function is prevented from operating, not because the critical neural system is completely useless, but because the compensation being utilized by other systems is preventing their operation. On Le Vere's model recovery and compensation are incompatible: if compensation is successful, then recovery of function cannot and will not take place. A primary effect of brain damage is a shift by the individual to undamaged systems. The aim of this process is to allow neural recovery by avoiding use of the lesioned tissue. However, while this would appear to be a useful strategy initially, the compensatory behaviours become established and recovery of the original behaviour is prevented following the neural recovery.

Le Vere has attempted to rationalize the unsatisfactory state of affairs which exists in the recovery of function area. He has drawn a clearer distinction between compensation and recovery, which by itself is not original, but his is the first attempt to explain recovery which incorporates the distinction in the model. An important feature of the model is that it redefines most of what we have considered to be recovery as compensation for lost behaviour. However, it is not entirely clear why lost (but recoverable) functions will not return following neural recovery when compensation has taken place. Le Vere has attempted to theorize only from an empirical database and has resisted the temptation to speculate beyond the evidence. The model is highly testable and has clear therapeutic implications.

LEFT HEMISPHERE INHIBITION OF RIGHT HEMISPHERE FUNCTION

The inhibition–facilitation dichotomy is fundamental to neurophysiology. It permeates all aspects of the field, providing powerful explanatory force at all levels, and forms the essential bedrock to our understanding of how the nervous system functions. Without it we would have no coherent theory of the nature of operation of the nervous system. The opposing forces of inhibition and facilitation or excitation are said to operate at the level of the cell, the synapse, and the neurotransmitters. For instance, at the synapse, the neurotransmitter acetyl choline is released to facilitate transmission across the synaptic gap and cholinesterase is released to neutralize the acetyl choline. The workings of the nervous system are explained in terms of this on/off, binary manner of operation. This powerful explanatory idea is also invoked at the level of mechanisms larger and more complex than the cell and synapse. Inhibition is an essential feature of the Jacksonian concept of *levels of representation*, where expression by lower levels is inhibited by higher controlling levels.

Moreover, the notion is also powerful in psychology, although it does not enjoy the same kind of scientific support. At a behavioural level, the operation of emotion, for example, is seen by many as being inhibited by cognition. Discussion in Chapter 5 showed that such a cognitivist characterization of the relationship between emotion and cognition—with cognition in control—is not supported by all those working in the field. The case has been made for influence operating in the opposite direction—affective mood-state influencing cognitive state.

Neuropsychology would appear to have inherited the notion of inhibition wholesale from neurology and applied it at what many would consider the 'highest' structural level—that of interaction between the hemispheres. Studies producing findings which cannot be accounted for in any other way often invoke some form of interhemispheric inhibition by way of explanation.

In interaction between the two sides of the brain, inhibition is usually seen to operate one-way—from left to right. The notion is the essential element of cerebral dominance theory, and a legacy of that theory. The left hemisphere dominates the right through the operation of often vaguely specified inhibitory forces of some kind. Such one-way interhemispheric inhibition is inconsistent with a fully complementary specialization model of hemispheric interaction. Not only is the notion not required, but it is conceptually inconsistent with the complementary specialization idea. Here the notion of interhemispheric inhibition becomes redundant unless it works both ways. That is to say, the right hemisphere must also have the capacity to inhibit the action of the left.

The notion of inhibition figures prominently in discussion of right hemisphere contributions to recovery in aphasia. The most interesting and controversial ideas to emerge in recent years are those of Moscovitch (1973, 1976) and Zaidel (1976, 1983). Moscovitch's (1973, 1976) 'functional localization model' of cerebral dominance for language was developed to reconcile what Moscovitch saw as contradictory accounts of neurolinguistic organization from the strict localization model (a strict left hemisphere characterization) and the split-brain model. The strict localization model derives its data from the massive literature on unilateral brain damage, which Moscovitch contrasts with the evidence from the commissurotomy studies. Moscovitch (1973) makes the point that both these databases are unsatisfactory foundations for a model of language organization in the normal brain:

> one cannot infer the functional organization of the cerebral hemispheres of normal people from studies conducted exclusively on brain-damaged individuals (p. 90).

The results of Moscovitch's (1972, 1973) reaction–time studies with normal subjects, referred to in an earlier chapter, suggested that the normal right hemisphere is superior for verbal material only when the task requires pictorial encoding but shows no ability when the task requires linguistic analysis. This lack of congruence between the normal right hemisphere (which showed no ability in his study), the separated and isolated right hemisphere, which, as we have seen, shows considerable linguistic abilities, and the linguistic performance of aphasic patients which, Moscovitch believes, falls short of what would be expected given split-brain and hemispherectomy evidence, forms the basis of his model. The functional localization model holds that the left hemisphere inhibits and suppresses right hemisphere language competence in the normal and aphasic brain via the corpus callosum, but inhibition cannot take place in split-brain and hemispherectomy patients, so inherent right hemisphere language abilities are released. The model suggests that the right hemisphere in both the normal and aphasic brain has abilities which are equal to the separated and isolated right hemisphere, but this capacity only becomes demonstrable when the left hemisphere is incapable of fulfilling its inhibitory role.

Moscovitch's model relies on three fundamental proposals: that the normal right hemisphere shows no linguistic capabilities; that the linguistic performance of aphasic patients is inferior to what is known about right hemisphere language in commissurotomy and hemispherectomy patients; and that many aphasic patients do not show any improvements in language functions. We will not repeat the findings discussed in detail in previous chapters which shows that there is substantial evidence for linguistic abilities in the normal right hemisphere. On the basis of the results of his studies on normal subjects, Day (1977) concluded that there is no inconsistency between the linguistic abilities of the separated and normal right hemisphere, and consequently, no requirement for an inhibition model to account for differences in right hemisphere abilities in the two groups.

The results of Zaidel's (1976, 1977) studies of separated and isolated right hemisphere performance on standardized tests of comprehension, also previously discussed in an earlier context (see Chapter 3), are inconsistent with the second assumption of Moscovitch's hypothesis. Zaidel's results indicate, if anything, the opposite: the right hemisphere in his subjects showed a severe deficit on the Token Test (mean MA 4 years) and aphasic patients, on average, perform slightly better. Performance on the Peabody and Ammons Picture Vocabulary tests was better than on the Token Test, with mean scores equivalent to a normal 11- to 12-year-old. This suggests that the auditory language comprehension of the right hemisphere in this population is no more than equivalent to that of an average aphasic performance. Zaidel (1976) concludes that:

> there is, on the average, no discrepancy between aphasia and commissurotomy data for auditory language comprehension and there are, therefore, no really competing models of right hemisphere auditory language comprehension to be reconciled. In particular there is no need to argue generally that left hemisphere control or inhibition masks right hemisphere language comprehension ability in the intact or left damaged brain (p. 206).

In addition, interpretation of the language abilities of the few adult hemispherectomy patients that have been examined may have been overestimated by Moscovitch, or at least there may be some error in perception of what constitutes an 'average' aphasic performance. After all, Zangwill's (1967) comments following his comprehensive examination of Smith's (1966) hemispherectomy patient, would indicate that the average aphasic patient's abilities are somewhat superior to that of an hemispherectomy patient:

> The general impression made upon me by this patient was very much like that of a case of *severe* [my italics] motor aphasia and right hemiplegia from left-sided cerebrovascular accident (p. 1017).

Moscovitch's third assumption concerning the absence of improvement in aphasic individuals must also be put into perspective. While it is undoubtedly the case that all too many aphasic patients do show marked and persisting impairments, a large proportion make excellent natural recoveries (Kertesz, 1979). Moreover, there are strong indications that a proportion of those patients who fail to make significant recovery have additional problems which have a material influence on prognosis. A number of studies have shown that the presence of ideomotor, ideational or constructional apraxia, or non-verbal intellectual impairment (Messorli, Tissot, and Rodriguez, 1976) or dysarthria (Gloning, Trappl, Heiss, and Quatember, 1976), for instance, have a significant negative effect on the degree of recovery in patients with aphasia. Recovery from aphasia can be hampered by additional factors which may also interfere with possible right hemisphere support of language. Moreover, the work that has shown that even global aphasic patients can make clinically, if not always statistically, significant recovery over as much as six years (Geschwind, 1974; Eisenson, 1981) suggests, firstly, that global aphasic patients may be capable of useful recovery, and also, may indicate a gradually developing right hemisphere capability. It would therefore appear that major differences in the comprehension abilities of these different groups may be more apparent than real, and more a function of our limited understanding of the complexity of the interactions involved.

As already mentioned, the notion of inhibition at the hemispheric level rests heavily on the concept of cerebral dominance. 'Inhibition' suggests an active controlling mechanism where the left hemisphere is almost consciously suppressing right hemisphere speech, when perhaps all that is required to fit more parsimoniously with the evidence is an 'interference' mechanism. It would appear, in some sense, to the inefficient, irrational, and not in the organism's best interests to allow a situation where a malfunctioning and ineffective system (the left hemisphere) is permitted to override a potentially effective back-up system. As Marshall and Patterson (1983) point out, the idea of a complete secondary system being developed only to be permanently inhibited by a dominant primary system is without parallel in biology.

The notion of inhibition, therefore, only becomes useful at the interhemispheric level if it is discrete and selective. If it is simply reactive, and works in an all-or-none fashion, it may best be characterized in terms of interference, but discrete inhibition could work positively to inhibit right hemisphere interference if left hemisphere mechanisms can achieve better results and be more effective in processing language. If, however, the site and degree of damage is such that left hemisphere control becomes impossible, then right hemisphere potential could be released from this discrete inhibition. This notion is in line with ideas expressed by Zaidel (Zaidel, 1976; Zaidel and Schweiger, 1984). Zaidel proposes a central mechanism (probably located in the left hemisphere) which regulates interhemispheric interaction. Zaidel and Schweiger speculate that left hemisphere lesions causing aphasia may compromise this mechanism to such an extent that it fails to release control to the right hemisphere.

With regard to the involvement of the right hemisphere in reading, Zaidel and Schweiger reason that the reading mechanisms of the two hemispheres are qualitatively different and thus a central controlling mechanism capable of intrahemispheric inhibition would be required to prevent, for example, the interference of a conflicting right hemisphere semantic specification with a left hemisphere semantic interpretation. On another occasion, the right-hemisphere-generated contribution might sometimes complement that of the left hemisphere to provide a full and rich specification. In such circumstances, the transfer of information from right to left hemisphere would be facilitated rather than inhibited. Zaidel and Schweiger here propose a form of inhibition which is discrete and includes some of the features of classical neurological inhibition (i.e., the dualism of inhibition and facilitation and the view that the left hemisphere is dominant in the sense that it is there that a control mechanism is probably located).

Alternatively, the control mechanism may rely on 'competence estimates' from the two hemispheres, and the damaged LH (especially with more posterior lesions) may provide distorted estimates, leading to the assignment of control to it, even when incompetent (Zaidel and Schweiger, 1984, p. 256).

Such a characterization fits well with the known 'optimistic' mood-state of many aphasic individuals with posterior damage. Although there is very little direct evidence for such a hypothesis at this stage, Zaidel and Schweiger have proposed a notion of interhemispheric inhibition which is more flexible and discriminatory than the all-or-none variety, and could have a complementary right hemisphere mechanism concerned with inhibition and facilitation of left hemisphere involvement in visuospatial processing. Left hemisphere inhibition of right hemisphere language competence may be inappropriate, especially in the severely damaged left hemisphere, 'so that speech may indeed occur in the right (non-dominant) hemisphere of some aphasics' (Zaidel, 1976, p. 209). Evidence reviewed earlier in this chapter supports this view: if shift takes place in aphasic patients, then the evidence suggests that it is in those who have severe aphasia. In more mildly affected patients, the left hemisphere may still be capable of sustaining language.

In the next chapter we turn to an examination of the evidence for the lateral shift hypothesis and find that ideas of recovery, sparing, and inhibition appear to figure variously in different conceptualizations of the hypothesis.

Chapter Seven

THE LATERAL SHIFT HYPOTHESIS: THE EVIDENCE

In this rather long chapter we examine the wide range of evidence in support of the lateral shift hypothesis. We first look at the sources of the evidence in turn, starting with the physiological evidence. We then turn our attention to the behavioural evidence, spending some time on the dichotic studies. Finally, we consider the evidence for right hemisphere involvement in aphasic symptomatology.

As indicated earlier, the hemispheric or lateral shift hypothesis has a long history. Broca (1865) observed recovery in cases of extensive left hemisphere damage which led him to suggest that in all probability the right hemisphere contributes to language comprehension and expression. We first consider the lesion cases which have been reported over the years. Some of these reports have had a marked influence on our conceptualizations of the role of the right hemisphere in aphasia.

LESION CASES

Gowers (1887), like Broca, also noted recovery following extensive damage to the third frontal convolution. Furthermore, he was probably the first to make the observation that right hemisphere activity must be involved in recovery in those cases where a subsequent right hemisphere lesion again produces aphasia:

> Loss of speech due to permanent destruction of the speech region in the left hemisphere has been recovered from, and that this recovery was due to supplemental action of the corresponding right hemisphere is proved by the fact that in some cases, speech has been again lost when a fresh lesion occurred in this part of the right hemisphere (Gowers, 1887, pp. 131–132).

Henschen (1922, cited by Nielsen, 1946) also argued for right hemisphere involvement in recovery from left hemisphere damage. In fact, the notion that the right hemisphere is responsible for recovery from aphasia was often referred to as 'Henschen's Axiom' (Kertesz, 1979). Henschen's arguments were also based on the observation, made earlier by Gowers and later extended by Neilsen (1946), that aphasia following left hemisphere damage could recover only to manifest again following a righ hemisphere lesion.

Neilsen (1946) studied a number of cases which led him to conclude:

the minor cerebral hemisphere assumes the function of the major in language with great facility in some instances, with great difficulty in others, and not at all in some persons (p. 155).

He further states that some functions may, while others may not, transfer:

the language function if partly destroyed does not usually transfer in toto; the visual, auditory or motor functions may be transferred separately (p. 155).

The cases described by Nielsen illustrate how the right hemisphere might take over the processing of functions compromised by a left hemisphere lesion, while apparently intact functions remain left hemisphere responsibilities.

Neilsen's cases include a right-handed female patient who suffered from a left hemisphere CVA causing right hemiplegia, Broca's aphasia, and moderate dysarthria. The patient apparently made a complete recovery, but nine years later she again became aphasic and hemiplegic (left) following a further CVA, this time to the right hemisphere. On the fourth day in hospital the patient died and autopsy confirmed old lesions in Broca's area on the left side and acute damage to the homogeneous area in the right hemisphere. Neilsen comments that (1946, p. 150) 'there can be no doubt that her speech for the nine years was carried on by the right motor speech area'.

A second case reported by Neilsen suggests that comprehension processes can shift to the right while expressive functions are still processed by the left hemisphere. This female patient suffered a left hemisphere CVA which rendered her aphasic. She rapidly recovered only to suffer a second left hemisphere CVA just four months later. The patient was said to understand speech, although totally unable to speak or write. The patient died and autopsy revealed an old lesion of the angular gyrus and the superior first temporal convolution as well as a recent lesion of Broca's area. Neilsen comments that the patient must have used the right temporal lobe for comprehension following the first stroke, and that was why comprehension remained intact following the second incident. However, the patient might have continued to use Broca's area on the left for expression following the first incident, otherwise she would not have become totally mute following the second lesion.

These kinds of case reports constitute strong clinical support for the hemispheric shift idea. Support comes also, however, from recent CT scan investigations of recovering global aphasic patients with extensive left hemisphere damage. Cummings, Benson, Walsh, and Levine (1979) present the case of a 54-year-old man who suffered a left CVA. Examination two months post-onset revealed a global aphasia with severe deficits in expression and comprehension. Re-examination three years later showed marked improvements in language functions, with comprehension showing the most improvement. CT scanning at this time showed:

a huge cystic area involving the entire middle cerebral artery distribution of the left hemisphere including all of the Broca's and Wernicke's areas plus a smaller infarct in the distribution of the right posterior cerebral artery (Cummings *et al.*, 1979, p. 1548).

The authors suggest that inferring right hemisphere responsibility for the marked recovery observed is inescapable. What is also of interest in this case is that comprehension was observed to have improved the most. Comprehension is known to improve more rapidly and more extensively than expression in the recovery of aphasia (Vignolo, 1964; Prins, Snow, and Wagenaar, 1978) and this may be due to right hemisphere involvement. A further study by this group (Landis, Cummings, and Benson, 1980) reports two cases of partial recovery arising very slowly in the evolution of global aphasia following what appears to be very extensive lesions of the left hemisphere encompassing all the classical language area. The authors comment that the linguistic recovery of the patients mirrored to some extent the linguistic capacities of the right hemisphere demonstrated in hemispherectomy and split-brain patients.

In a CT scan study, Pieniadz, Naeser, Koff, and Levine (1983) examined the relationships between hemispheric asymmetries (width and length) and recovery in 14 global aphasic patients by comparing asymmetries to 60 normal controls and 89 aphasic patients. The globally impaired patients were assessed at 1 to 7 months ('T1') and again at 7 to 30 months ('T2') on a range of tests. All patients had extensive left hemisphere lesions including frontal, parietal, temporal, and subcortical damage. No significant relationships were found between test scores and age, months post-onset or lesion size. What the study did find was that patients who scored higher on tests at T2 and showed most improvement between T1 and T2 (particularly in comprehension, repetition and naming, all at the one-word level) exhibited the most marked atypical asymmetries on the scans, especially in the occipital region.

The authors note that it was atypical posterior asymmetries which correlated with language impairments usually associated with posterior lesions and draw parallels with right hemisphere linguistic abilities in commissurotomy subjects. Specifically, one-word level processing ability, greater ability in 'posterior' language functions, and poor speech processing.

> Perhaps the right hemisphere, in the 'recovered' global aphasia cases with atypical asymmetries, can aid in language recovery by complementing or cooperating with the few preserved areas of the left hemisphere in some unique manner not ordinarily utilized by 'unrecovered' global aphasia cases with typical asymmetries (Pieniadz *et al.*, 1983, pp. 388–389).

SOME CEREBRAL BLOODFLOW EVIDENCE

In Chapter 2 we examined the application of this technique (rCBF) to the hemispheric differences field. The technique has not been widely applied to aphasic subjects. One study (Yamaguchi, Meyer, Sakai, and Yamamoto, 1980) has reported on rCBF results for three aphasic patients and offers some support for the hemispheric shift idea. In one patient with severe Broca's aphasia due to bilateral occlusion of the middle cerebral arteries, rCBF measures revealed essentially normal resting values in the right and reduction of activity in the left hemisphere. During psychophysical activation (counting, speaking, watching, listening to music) bloodflow was bilaterally decreased. Subsequently a bypass operation was performed between the left middle cerebral and left superficial temporal arteries. Some improvement was observed in aphasia following this and further rCBF measures three months later showed no increase of bloodflow in Broca's area but an increase of 20% in the homologous area in the right hemisphere.

The second patient was aphasic secondary to a left middle cerebral artery embolic occlusion. This patient underwent left carotid endarterectomy and made a good recovery so that his problems were fairly mild at the time of rCBF testing. Resting mean rCBF values were low normal; during psychophysical activation increase in left hemisphere rCBF was lower than in normal subjects but right hemisphere values were essentially normal. An 8% increase in the right hemisphere Broca's area was also observed. The third case in this series had a 'mixed' aphasia following coronary bypass surgery. He made an excellent recovery and his language was described as normal unless fatigued. Resting rCBF values were normal in both hemispheres and increased normally during activation.

Yamaguchi et al. interpret these results to suggest the possibility that the right hemisphere becomes involved in patients with good recovery.

THE SODIUM AMYTAL EVIDENCE

The sodium amytal evidence, such as it is, tends to support other data which indicate that for some individuals the right brain can support some recovery from aphasia. One or two sodium amytal studies only have addressed themselves to the investigation of hemispheric shift in aphasic patients. Kinsbourne (1971) tested three right-handed male patients who were all aphasic secondary to left hemisphere damage. The first case had made some recovery by six weeks post-onset, being able to imitate consonant sounds although vowels were distorted. Although able to articulate a number of single words recognizably, he was unable to speak in phrases. Comprehension was reported to be relatively unimpaired. During right intracarotid injection (right hemisphere anaesthesia):

> the patient was totally unable to phonate or even to move his tongue and lips to command. Afterwards he reported that he had tried to speak, knew which words he wanted to use, but found himself unable to exert control over his speech musculature.

During left intracarotid injection (left hemisphere anaesthesia), on the other hand, the patient:

could phonate, move tongue and lips to command and respond verbally in recognizable fashion (Kinsbourne, 1971, p. 303).

In addition, although verbal perseveration had not previously been a characteristic of the patient's aphasia, he tended to perseverate on his own name during left hemisphere anaesthesia.

The expressive abilities of Kinsbourne's second patient were also severely compromised with comprehension being relatively unimpaired. Kinsbourne describes the patient as a conduction aphasic patient, being slow and often incorrect at repeating single and paired digits. No other details are given on the patient's deficits. During right hemisphere anaesthesia this patient was also unable to phonate or move his tongue and lips to command. Like the first patient, he reported afterwards that he knew what he wanted to say but was unable to formulate the words. With left hemisphere anaesthesia expressive abilities were unaffected, except that he gave some associative responses to the digits he was asked to repeat—something he normally did not do.

The third patient in Kinsbourne's study was described as a globally affected patient with poor comprehension and expression. He was able to produce some single words, but there was a severe deficit in confrontation naming. This patient received only left hemisphere sodium amytal anaesthesia which did not affect his ability to name objects or comprehend commands.

There would appear to be some problems with Kinsbourne's cases in so far as their difficulties under right hemisphere anaesthesia could have been due simply to induced dysarthria. A complete inability to phonate or to move the lips and tongue sounds very much more like a neuromuscular paralysis than it does apraxia of speech. A severe pseudobulbar palsy-type of dysarthria requires bilateral upper motor neurone lesions, and right hemisphere anaesthesia on top of a left hemisphere lesion may have induced such a condition in these patients. The problem is that Kinsbourne's description of subjects' impairments under hemispheric anaesthesia does not rule out dysarthria.

It appears as if left hemisphere anaesthesia induces some reportedly slight expressive disorders (perseveration in one patient and 'associative responses' to digits in another) in the aphasic patients tested. Even if we ignore the right hemisphere anaesthesia evidence on the grounds that 'aphasic speech' could not be assessed in subjects who may have been totally anarthric, then we are left only with the left hemisphere anaesthesia data. The subjects' responses during left hemisphere anaesthesia suggest that very little of the patients' language ability required the unanaesthetized processing capacity of the left hemisphere. That is to say, the sodium amytal evidence, such as it is, suggests that hemispheric shift can take place in global aphasic patients.

A larger sodium amytal study has recently been reported in English by Czopf (1979) although originally published in German (Czopf, 1972). Czopf subjected 30 patients to sodium amytal injection and reported on 22. Something has evidently been lost in translation of this paper is it is difficult to determine the actual numbers of vascular compared to trauma patients or the severity of some of the subgroups. However, right hemisphere anaesthesia in 10 of the aphasic subjects (time since onset ranges from 3 weeks to 13 years) was reported to produce very severe deficits in language functions. Left hemisphere anaesthesia in just two of these patients affected speech to a lesser degree and for a shorter period than with right hemisphere anaesthesia. In three of the group right-sided injection had no effect on language functions 'although it elicited signs of loss of hemisphere control' (Czopf, 1979, p. 28). What 'loss of hemispheric control' means is not actually clear. These three patients had mild aphasia of very recent onset (2, 10, and 14 days) and left-sided injection in one of the patients produced a severe aphasia.

In a further subgroup (the numbers are uncertain) aphasia was apparently moderately worsened with injection of either side. Czopf (1979) concludes that:

> speech deterioration following temporary obliteration of right hemisphere function was extensive in those cases whose aphasia had originally been severe and had been present for a long period of time. One might assume, therefore, that the degree of substitution by the non-dominant hemisphere is positively correlated with time (p. 29).

Brown (1979) has observed (but has not reported details) that in his experience right hemisphere anaesthesia may have different effects depending on the type of aphasia. In one conduction aphasic patient left-sided injection had little effect on performance but right-sided injection produced severe phonemic paraphasia. In a jargon patient injection on either side had no effect.

The scanty sodium amytal evidence must be interpreted with care. It appears as if some of the deficits following right-sided injection in patients who already have a left hemisphere lesion, may be the result of an induced pseudobulbar palsy. This interpretation, applied to the well-reported responses of Kinsbourne's subjects, probably applies also to the cases reported by Czopf. Bearing this proviso in mind, the evidence suggests that right hemisphere participation in language functions following left hemisphere damage depends on severity of aphasia, time since onset of aphasia and, maybe, type of aphasia. Some patients show no evidence of right hemisphere participation at all—those who have mild aphasia of recent onset.

ELECTROENCEPHALOGRAPHY

Finally in this section we turn to electroencephalography (EEG). The technique has not been used extensively to examine the claims of the hemispheric shift hypothesis. Those studies which have been completed tend to support the hypothesis (Tikofsky, Kooi, and Thames, 1960; Moore, 1984). Tikofsky *et al.* found that patients with abnormal EEG patterns over the left hemisphere showed improvement in language whereas those with abnormal tracings over both hemispheres showed no improvement in language. Recently, an interesting study by Moore has compared left and right EEG patterns in 12 aphasic, 12 normal male, and 12 normal female subjects. Five of the aphasic subjects were non-fluent and 7 were fluent. Time since onset ranged from 1 year to 29 years (mean 7.6 years) and the mean age of the aphasic group was 54.8 years. Subjects were required to imitate 10 sentences and answer 10 questions on a story that was read to them ('yes/no' or 'true/false' responses) while EEG measures were taken. Subjects who were not able to complete significant amounts of the tasks were excluded from the study.

Looking at the amount of alpha that subjects were producing only during stimulus presentation, and the number of correct responses on the comprehension task and correct repetitions on the imitation task, Moore found that the aphasic subjects showed greater alpha suppression on the right hemisphere for both the comprehension and repetition tasks.

> This suggests that subjects who have sustained known left cerebral brain insult, with subsequent language disturbances, become more reliant on right hemisphere processing strategies when processing linguistic material (Moore, 1984, p. 202).

Additionally, no differences were found between fluent and non-fluent patients, suggesting to Moore that both non-fluent and fluent aphasic patients use the right hemisphere to more or less the same degree. There was also significantly more suppression of alpha over the right hemisphere in fluent and non-fluent patients while engaged on the repetition task than during the comprehension task. However, as Moore concedes, the normal females also showed greater alpha suppression on the comprehension task and four of the aphasic subjects were female (three of whom were fluent). It may be that the results reflect a sex difference in the aphasic subjects.

THE DICHOTIC LISTENING EVIDENCE

As indicated in Chapter 2, dichotic listening has proved a popular method in neuropsychological research. It has been widely used as a comparatively simple, non-invasive technique for determining 'hemispheric' advantage or preference for particular auditory materials or processes through ear advantages or preferences. In this section we will be concerned with studies which have examined the dichotic performance of aphasic patients. A number of studies have found left ear advantages for verbal materials in aphasic groups and individuals which have been interpreted as evidence for a shift to the right hemisphere for language processing. Unfortunately, other interpretations indicate that hemispheric preference cannot be reliably determined with dichotic listening in brain damaged individuals. Essentially, studies group into those which have interpreted results in terms of a 'dominance effect' and those which have identified a 'lesion effect'. A variety of stimulus materials, response methods, and types have been employed, not all of which may be appropriate for use with severely impaired subjects.

Moore and Weidner (1975) examined the dichotic results of 30 aphasic subjects and 10 controls using a 24-pair CVC dichotic word test made up of rhyming word pairs (e.g., 'mat–bat') which was used with a multiple-choice picture-pointing response method. The control group obtained a significantly higher right ear score and significantly lower left ear score than any of three aphasic onset subgroups. No significant differences were found between the mean dichotic performances of the three aphasic subgroups, although there was a trend towards increased left ear scores with increased time since onset. Moore and Weidner suggested that these results indicate that there is not simply a decrement in the ear scores of aphasic patients, but a clear shift to a left ear (right hemisphere) preference. This shift to the right hemisphere, they suggest, increases as a function of time post-onset.

Johnson, Sommers, and Weidner (1977) examined the relationships between dichotic performance and initial severity of aphasia as determined by assessment within the first four weeks post-onset. The 20 right-handed aphasic subjects (10 male and 10 female) all suffered posterior left hemisphere damage and were grouped into less than six months post-onset and more than six months post-onset. The test used in this study was a slightly modified version of the simple CVC rhyming test used by Moore and Weidner. Group analysis revealed a significant left ear advantage for the aphasic group and a significant right ear advantage for controls. Although no significant interactions were observed between dichotic results and time since onset, a greater left ear advantage was obtained by subjects of more than six months post-onset than subjects of less than six months post-onset. Initial severity of aphasia appeared to influence significantly the dichotic performance of subjects. Those subjects who initially had mild/moderate language problems produced a significantly smaller left ear advantage than patients initially assessed to have moderate/marked problems. J.P. Johnson *et al.* suggest that their results indicate a shift to the right hemisphere in aphasic patients, with a greater reliance on the right hemisphere in the more severely aphasic.

Brady (1978) also examined the relationships between severity of aphasia and ear preferences in 15 subjects, aphasic secondary to posterior left hemisphere damage, all of early onset (one to three months), using the same dichotic test as J. P. Johnson *et al.* Results agreed essentially with those obtained by J. P. Johnson *et al.* The 'severe' subgroup (there were five subjects in each subgroup) showed a larger left ear advantage then the 'moderate' subgroup, with the 'mild' subgroup producing a right ear advantage approximately equivalent to that produced by the control group.

In their study, Pettit and Noll (1979) attempted to measure dichotic performance and recovery in aphasia. They administered a dichotic digit and a dichotic animal-name test together with aphasia tests on two occasions two months apart to 25 unselected subjects. Dichotic pairs were presented in groups of three and subjects were allowed a choice of response mode, including oral report, writing, or pointing to animal pictures or numbers made from felt. Retest on the aphasia assessment revealed a significant mean improvement in scores for the aphasic group as a whole, although there was a great deal of individual variability. Significant differences were observed between the right ear advantage obtained by the control group and the left ear advantage produced by the aphasic group. In addition, on dichotic retest for the aphasic subjects, there was a significant reduction in mean errors for the left ear on the digit and animal-name tests, but not for the right ear. So as language abilities improved over a two-month period, there was an accompanying improvement in left ear performance. Pettit and Noll's (1979, p. 197) conclusion was that this constituted 'strong evidence for the argument that a shift in dominance occurs as the aphasic improves in language ability'.

There have been one or two studies comparing the dichotic performances of different clinical types of aphasia. Crosson and Warren (1981) compared 12 normal, 8 Wernicke's, and 12 Broca's subjects using the identical CVC test used by J. P. Johnson et al. and Brady and the same picture-pointing multiple-choice response method. The Wernicke's and Broca's groups both produced a left ear advantage compared to the normal group, but although the Wernicke's group showed a larger left ear preference than the Broca's group, the difference was not significant.

A large retrospective and longitudinal study has examined the dichotic peformance of 117 aphasic patients classified as fluent or non-fluent and tested on up to three dichotic tests (Castro-Caldas and Botelho, 1980). The tests were a 34-pair object–word test involving a picture-pointing response, a 19-pair digit test requiring oral report, and an 18-pair word test also requiring oral report. The retrospective study involved dividing the sample into those subjects who were tested within six months post-onset and those tested after six months post-onset. Non-fluent subjects showed a significant tendency towards a left ear preference on retest with the 18-pair word test, whereas fluent patients showed a significant tendency towards a right ear advantage on retest on both the 18- and 34-word-pair tests.

The longitudinal study entailed testing a sample of patients twice within 12 months. Results showed an increase in right ear preference on retest for fluent subjects on the two word tests. Castro-Caldas and Botelho (1980, p. 150) suggest that their results indicate 'a relative functional ambidominance of the neural structures responsible for verbal decoding'. These structures, they state, are controlled through anterior mechanisms which are also responsible for verbal encoding. An anterior lesion resulting in a non-fluent aphasia causes imbalance in this system and results in anterior right hemisphere takeover.

This homologous anterior right hemisphere structure takes on control of the posterior decoding system, which is what underlies the shift in hemispheric dominance reflected in the left ear preference on dichotic testing. In subjects with fluent aphasia the anterior system is undamaged and still in control of the sensory cortex. The left hemisphere remains dominant for language in fluent aphasic patients, and a tendency towards a right ear preference will therefore be observed, especially at later stages post-onset.

Castro-Caldas and Botelho's (1980) model ignores the contrary evidence from other investigations and, like some other dichotic studies with brain damaged subjects, fails to take into account the 'lesion effect'.

The lesion effect

The studies reviewed above have interpreted results to reflect clear hemispheric preference. Other dichotic studies with brain damaged patients suggest that this is too simplistic an interpretation and that the effects of the lesion on ear preferences must be taken into account.

The inference of hemispheric advantage from ear advantage on dichotic tests assumes the integrity of an individual's entire auditory system, including the primary auditory cortex and association cortex of both left and right hemispheres, and the interconnecting commissural pathways linking the association cortices in both temporal lobes. Damage to any part of this area, at least, can give rise to a 'lesion effect' on dichotic results. A number of studies have identified the lesion effect in the performance of brain damaged subjects and separated it from the 'dominance effect' (Kimura, 1961; Milner, 1962; Sparks and Geschwind, 1968; Milner, Taylor, and Sperry, 1968; Schulhoff and Goodglass, 1969). The lesion effect tends to result in an impairment, suppression or total extinction of stimuli in the ear contralateral to the lesion, whereas the dominance effect produces the expected higher scores in the ear contralateral to the hemisphere specialized in processing the material or tasks that the dichotic test is being used to assess. Stated another way,

> the 'lateral dominance effect' is a function of the stimulus used, while the 'lesion effect' represents the disadvantage to the contralateral ear, regardless of material used (Schulhoff and Goodglass, 1969, p. 154).

Schulhoff and Goodglass (1969) analysed the performance of a control, a left-hemisphere-damaged group, and a right-hemisphere-damaged group on a variety of dichotic tasks. There were verbal tests consisting of two, three, and four sets of digits for oral report, a 'right hemisphere' musical task consisting of two-note and three-note sequences requiring a non-verbal response, and a 'neutral' dichotic click task requiring an oral report. The left hemisphere group were reported to have mild/moderate aphasia, but site of lesion (anterior or posterior) or type of aphasia was not reported. Controls produced the expected preferences, but for the brain damaged groups, Schulhoff and Goodglass found a bilateral decrement in performance on material for which the damaged hemisphere was specialized. For the left-brain-damaged subjects, group results showed a non-significant right ear superiority for digits (4.2%), although 6 of the 10 subjects actually showed a left ear·advantage. These subjects produced a 'normal' left ear advantage on the music test, the group scores being almost identical to the control group's mean ear-preference scores on the music test. On the neutral click-counting task the left hemisphere group produced a significant left ear advantage. The results for the right hemisphere group paralleled the findings for the left hemisphere group in some respects. There was bilateral decrement for digits as compared with controls, but a clear right ear superiority. There was also a bilateral decrement for music, but a left ear preference was maintained and click-counting revealed a bilateral decrement also, with a non-significant right ear advantage. These group results support a lesion effect explanation, although results for individual subjects, especially on the digit task, showed much variability.

The lesion effect was further investigated by Sparks, Goodglass, and Nickel (1970) in 28 left-hemisphere-damaged and 20 right-hemisphere-damaged subjects, all of 'recent onset'. No information was provided on type of degree of aphasia or localization of lesion. A two-pair digit and single-pair animal name test requiring oral report were used. Both brain damaged groups produced a decrement in the ear contralateral to the side of injury for digits and words. The results not only provide further support for the lesion effect hypothesis, but also provide evidence for the notion that dichotically presented verbal information travels from left ear to right hemisphere and thence to left hemisphere via the corpus callosum, and from right ear to left hemisphere via the contralateral auditory pathways.

The evidence for this comes from the left hemisphere group which consisted of subjects exhibiting either contralateral right ear or 'paradoxical' left ear suppression, whereas the right-hemisphere group exhibited only contralateral suppression. Left hemisphere lesions, on Sparks *et al.*'s interpretation, can impede dichotic stimuli arriving at the left auditory cortex from the left ear via the right hemisphere and the corpus callosum, and from the right ear via the contralateral auditory pathway. Right brain lesions, on the other hand, can only affect stimuli from the left ear as the contralateral pathway from right ear to the left temporal lobe is unaffected by the right hemisphere lesion. A diagrammatic representation of the model proposed by Sparks *et al.* is presented in Figure 5.

Some left-hemisphere-damaged aphasic patients show a left ear advantage and others a right ear advantage on dichotic tests involving the processing of verbal material. Why this is so was examined further by Shanks and Ryan (1976) who tested 11 randomly selected aphasic patients and 11 matched controls. Time since onset ranged from 1 to 45 months and there was a variety of aetiologies. A 30-pair CV syllable test was used where subjects could either record responses orally or through pointing. The study produced some interesting findings. Although both groups produced a right ear preference, six of the aphasic group produced a right ear and five a left ear advantage. Shanks and Ryan comment that the group analysis tended 'to neutralize or obscure the performances of the two distinct aphasic subgroups' (p. 108). The study found no relationships between severity or time since onset, but this was hardly surprising bearing in mind the small size of the sample and the large range in onset times.

Dichotic listening with brain damaged subjects has been extended in recent

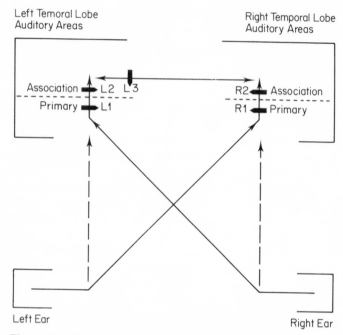

Left Temoral Lobe
Auditory Areas

Right Temporal Lobe
Auditory Areas

Association — L2 L3

R2 — Association

Primary — L1

R1 — Primary

Left Ear

Right Ear

Figure 5   Model proposed by Sparks, Goodglass, and Nickel (1970) to explain extinction of dichotic stimuli in brain damaged patients. The broken lines represent the ipsilateral pathways and the areas L1, L2, L3, R1, R2 represent the sites of lesions which can produce extinction. From Sparks, Goodglass, and Nickel (1970). Ipsilateral versus contralateral extinction in dichotic listening resulting from hemispheric lesions. *Cortex*, **6**, 249–260.

studies with the aim of looking at its potential for anatomical study rather than laterality study. Damasio and Damasio (1979) conducted a study with the primary aim of mapping the course of the interhemispheric auditory pathways by comparing ear preferences with actual lesion sites. Twenty brain-damaged subjects who had had CT scans were split into three groups on the basis of their ear-preference scores. A 'left ear extinction' group consisted of those subjects who obtained a laterality quotient of +14 or more, a 'right ear extinction' group were those who obtained a laterality quotient of −10 or more (+ denotes a right ear advantage and − a left ear advantage), and those who obtained scores between these two figures were considered as having produced a 'normal' dichotic performance. Left ear extinction was noted to be associated with lesions in the left and right posterior parieto-occipital and midtemporal regions. Right ear extinction, on the other hand, was related to lesions in the left temporal and the right parieto-occipital regions. Subjects who obtained 'normal' ear scores had lesions in the right frontal, left frontal, and left posterior occipital regions. Damasio and Damasio conclude that left ear extinction is caused by a lesion at any point along the course of the interhemispheric auditory pathway, irrespective of hemisphere, which, they argue, must run from the geniculo-cortical pathways posteriorly and upwards to arch around the lateral ventricles joining the posterior region of the corpus callosun.

Finally, Niccum, Rubens, and Speaks (1981) compared the performance of 16 aphasic subjects on a range of verbal dichotic tasks. Subjects averaged three years post-onset and were described as mildly aphasic. The tests used were made up of either digits, high-contrast words (e.g., pie, tree, cloud), vowel words (e.g., key, cow, car), consonant-words (e.g., pan, fan, man), or CV syllables. The digit, high-contrast, and vowel-words tests produced essentially identical patterns of performance in the 16 subjects; viz., a significant left ear advantage with low right ear scores. The consonant-words test produced lower left ear and right ear scores, but still produced a significant left ear advantage. Performance dropped markedly on the CV syllable test. Examination of CT scan results showed that subjects could be split into those who achieved right ear scores in excess of 75% of those with right ear scores less than 50% on the digit test. The former had intact primary auditory cortex and geniculo-temporal pathways suggesting spared auditory processing mechanisms, while the latter had lesions extending into primary auditory cortex.

Also of interest was the finding that the consonant-words test (the one most similar to the test used in the early studies with aphasic patients) had the advantage of being highly sensitive to lesions and more susceptible to lesion effects, even, perhaps to small lesions outside the geniculo-temporal systems. The CV syllable test has serious limitations as a clinical tool due to the high proportion of errors obtained even in non-dichotic binaural conditions. The authors point out, furthermore, that even normal subjects produce high error rates on CV syllable tests.

Before we summarize this section on the role of dichotic listening in the study of hemispheric shift in aphasic patients, we look at the relevance of phonetic or stimulus dominance effects observed in responses on dichotic tests with brain damaged patients.

Phonetic preferences of brain damaged subjects on dichotic tests

In the discussion on dichotic listening in Chapter 2 we described how the ear advantages observed in dichotic studies were to some extent determined by the phonetic characteristics of the stimuli. We will not repeat this here, but essentially, the general finding is that normal subjects show a preference for voiceless over voiced stops, for velar place over alveolar place of articulation, and for alveolar over bilabial place of articulation.

Several investigations have shown that left-hemisphere-damaged aphasic subjects tend to exhibit greater impairment in discriminating phonemes contrasting in place of articulation than phonemes contrasting in presence or absence of voice and that this effect influences the choices that aphasic subjects make on dichotic tests (Oscar-Berman, Zurif, and Blumstein, 1975; Blumstein, Baker, and Goodglass, 1977; Miceli, Caltagirione, Gainotti, and Payer-Rigo, 1978). What is of particular relevance for the main question posed in this chapter is that the choices made by aphasic subjects on the basis of phonetic features may involve more right than left hemisphere processing.

The phonetic preferences of 16 unilaterally left-hemisphere-damaged and 9 right-hemisphere-damaged subjects on a synthetic CV syllable test have been analysed by Oscar-Berman et al. (1975). Information is not provided on the handedness of the subjects or how many of the left-hemisphere-damaged were aphasic, but it is implied that most had some mild degree of aphasia. Group analysis showed that subjects identified significantly more syllables heard in the ear ipsilateral to the side of injury than in the ear contralateral to the side of injury. Left-hemisphere-damaged subjects reported significantly more left ear syllables than either the control or right-hemisphere-damaged group.

Analysis of the phonetic characteristics of correctly identified stimuli showed interesting differences between groups. For dichotic pairs which did not share either the features voice or place (for instance /p/ and /g/, which are initial phonemes that have maximum phonetic contrast within the class of stop, with /p/ being a voiceless bilabial and /g/ being a voiced velar stop), no real differences were found between groups. For syllable pairs which shared phonetic features, however (for instance /b/ and /g/, both being voiced, or /t/ and /d/ both sharing alveolar place), the performance of the left hemisphere group was significantly worse than that of the controls. Controls benefited most from shared place and less from shared voice; a result which supports the general finding of other studies (Studdert-Kennedy, Shankweiler, and Pisoni, 1972; Allen and Haggard, 1977). The most interesting finding, however, was that the left hemisphere group's error rate was much lower when two competing syllables shared voice than when two syllables shared place or shared no features. Figure 6.3 from Oscar-Berman et al. (1975) shows that although the left hemisphere group failed to profit from any feature sharing, there was a significant advantage in their ability to use the feature voice. The right hemisphere group were also able to use voice over place, but the difference was below significance.

The authors interpret the left-hemisphere-damaged subjects' ability to take advantage of shared voice and not shared place as being due to the acoustic rather than the phonetic basis of the feature voice. They argue that the dimension of voice onset time, one of the primary dimensions distinguishing voiced from voiceless stops, is mainly perceivable from acoustic parameters and relies mostly on temporal analysis. The feature place, in contrast, has been shown to be more phonetically encoded and perception appears to depend on spectral analysis. It is when the linguistic features of dichotic stimuli are more easily obtainable from such acoustic parameters, rather than from phonetic ones, that the performance of left-hemisphere-damaged subjects improves. This non-phonetic processing strategy utilized by subjects with compromised left hemisphere phonetic processing systems may conceivably involve right hemisphere acoustic processing.

Summary

In the search for relationships between various aphasic variables and ear scores on dichotic tests results have been inconclusive. This may be due in part to fairly loose subject selection criteria as well as to different interpretations of the results. Some studies have found correlations between increased left ear scores and severity of aphasia (J. P. Johnson *et al.*, 1977; Brady, 1978) while Pettit and Noll (1979) found an increase in left ear scores with improvement in aphasia test scores in their longitudinal study. Some studies have found significant increases in left ear advantage with increased time since onset (Moore and Weidner, 1975; Pettit and Noll, 1979) while others have found no such relationship (J. P. Johnson *et al.*, 1977). It would appear that aphasic subjects can be split into two distinct groups: those who produce a right ear advantage and those who produce a left ear advantage (Schulhoff and Goodglass, 1969; Shanks and Ryan, 1976; Damasio and Damasio, 1979; Castro-Caldas and Botelho, 1980; Crosson and Warren, 1981). Castro-Caldas and Botelho observed that fluent posterior patients increased their right ear scores over time whereas non-fluent anterior patients increased their left ear scores. In contrast, Crosson and Warren (1981), who simply compared the ear-preference scores of Wernicke's and Broca's patients, found that the former had the larger left ear advantage, although the difference was insignificant.

It is clear from the foregoing review that the major issue facing dichotic listening research with aphasic subjects is the extent to which it is possible to divorce the influence on results of a dominance from a lesion effect. How much credence can be given to the claim that an ear preference reflects a hemispheric preference in brain damage patients? Correlations between severity of aphasia and increased left ear scores can unfortunately be explained satisfactorily in terms of the lesion effect. Both J. P. Johnson *et al.*'s (1977) and Brady's (1978) subjects, for instance, had left temporo-parietal damage and Damasio and Damasio's (1979) findings indicate that ear preferences in patients with damage to this region are due to a lesion effect and a hemispheric shift for linguistic processing cannot be justifiably inferred. Larger brain lesions will generally produce more severe aphasia, and a larger and denser lesion will probably yield a greater reduction in right ear scores. Thus, severity of aphasia and extinction of a right ear advantage in posterior patients may be seen as dual, direct, functions of extent of lesion. It may not therefore be possible to separate out the influence of the lesion effect from the dominance effect on ear perferences in aphasic patients with posterior damage.

There is some evidence, however, which suggests that dichotic listening may still have a role to play in investigations into hemispheric shift in aphasic patients. Given that the lesion effect can account for the correlations reported between dichotic performance and severity, it is unable to account in any clear and direct way for the increase in left ear scores as an apparent function of time since onset (Moore and Weidner, 1975; Pettit and Noll, 1979). Damasio and Damasio's results, for instance, do not answer the question as to why patients with non-fluent aphasia due to an anterior lesion, but presumably with preserved left auditory association cortex, should show a left ear advantage, as left ear extinction in their study was associated with lesions in the left and right parieto-occipital and right midtemporal regions. On the available evidence, therefore, the non-fluent aphasic patient who produces a left ear advantage, with intact posterior speech processing mechanisms and interhemispheric callosal pathway from right to left auditory cortex, is demonstrating a genuine dominance effect—a lateral shift to the right hemisphere for auditory verbal processing. On our current understanding of the influence of lesion and dominance effects on dichotic scores. a comparison of ear scores in fluent and non-fluent aphasic patients at early and later stages of onset should show an increase in left ear scores in non-fluent subjects over time—indicating increased processing in the right hemisphere, but a maintenance of ear-preference scores in fluent patients—reflecting a lesion effect.

Such an interpretation of the current lesion and dominance effect models formed the basis for a recent study (Code, 1983a). Twenty-seven aphasic subjects grouped into fluent (posterior) and non-fluent (anterior) were tested on a rhyming CVC word test like that used by J. P. Johnson et al. (1977) and Brady (1978). Significantly higher left ear scores were found in non-fluent subjects who were more than 12 months post-onset than in non-fluents who were less than 12 months post-onset. In addition, right ear scores were found to be significantly lower in non-fluents of more than 12 months post-onset when compared to non-fluents of less than 12 months post-onset. No significant differences were found, however, between the ear scores of fluent subjects at less than and more than 12 months post-stroke.

Although the study was not a longitudinal one, was conducted on a relatively small group of subjects, and used only one short dichotic test, the results suggest that for fluent subjects with damaged posterior speech processing mechanisms, dichotic performance reflects a lesion effect which cannot be reliably interpreted in terms of hemispheric shift. For non-fluent patients with undamaged posterior mechanisms, the findings may suggest an increasing involvement of the right hemisphere in speech processing—a dominance effect.

The intimate functional relationships which probably exist between anterior and posterior language mechanisms should not be ignored, however: a lesion in anterior regions could very easily interfere with processing in the posterior areas. None the less, the results of Damasio and Damasio would suggest that lesions outside the primary auditory processing areas and pathways do not interfere significantly with dichotic performance. It is hoped that future studies will examine in further detail the relationships between anatomical damage, dichotic performance, and recovery from aphasia.

FURTHER SUPPORTIVE EVIDENCE FROM BEHAVIOURAL STUDIES

There appear to have been few investigations into the question of hemispheric shift in aphasic patients using other behavioural techniques for determining 'lateralization'. What studies have been completed are examined in this short section. Why there have been so few tachistoscopic studies is not entirely clear. The method is not expensive or technically complex and, despite the problems of interpretation of findings discussed in Chapter 2, is reasonably reliable and non-invasive. The reason researchers have tended to avoid the technique with brain damaged subjects is probably because of the presence of visual-field defects and—especially with right-hemisphere-damaged— unilateral neglect in many patients.

Shai, Goodglass, and Barton (1972) tested 10 left-hemisphere-damaged and 10 right-hemisphere-damaged subjects and 10 controls on a verbal (15 high frequency three-letter words) and a non-verbal (15 nonsense figures) unilateral tachistoscopic task. Left hemisphere patients produced significantly higher left visual-field scores for both types of material, while right hemisphere patients obtained significantly better right visual-field scores for both verbal and non-verbal materials.

Moore and Weidner (1974) tested 30 aphasic patients on a bilateral verbal tachistoscopic task employing high frequency rhyming CVC word pairs. A control group produced a right visual-field advantage for the task, whereas the aphasic group produced a significant left visual-field advantage. Moore and Weidner examined the possible influence of time since onset but no significant interaction between visual-field preferences and this variable was observed. A dominance effect interpretation of the results of these two studies would suggest a shift to the right hemisphere for language processing in the left-hemisphere-damaged patient with a shift to the left for processing nonsense shapes in right-hemisphere-damaged patients. This pattern of results, however, also raises the question of lesion effects influencing the visual-field preferences of brain damaged subjects.

The time-sharing paradigm has recently been used with aphasic patients. This method would appear, on the face of it, to avoid some of the problems of other tests of lateralization. With this technique, disruption of hand tapping during language tasks is taken to indicate left hemisphere processing for language with right hand disturbance and right hemisphere processing for language with left hand disruption. Mixed hand-tapping disturbance is said to indicate bilateral representation for language. The theoretical basis for the paradigm is discussed in Chapter 2.

Klingman and Sussman (1983) report results for eight Broca's aphasics compared to eight normal subjects using the time-sharing technique. They measured left and right hand tapping while subjects completed expressive and receptive verbal tasks. Controls produced higher right hand (left hemisphere) interference indicating left hemisphere specialization for the experimental tasks. In contrast, group results showed that the Broca's patients produced a highly symmetrical disturbance pattern, suggested by the paradigm to indicate bilateral processing during the experimental tasks. No interactions were found between laterality scores and either Boston Exam performance, or CT scans available for four of the patients. However, individual performance was highly variable. One patient appeared to show evidence for right hemisphere processing of expression during testing, and four for reception only. Only two patients (8 and 1) produced sufficiently asymmetric scores to indicate right hemisphere processing during both expressive and receptive tasks.

Subject 1 was a 24-year-old whose CT scan showed frontal and anterior temporal lobe damage due to a gunshot wound some 2 years 7 months earlier. Patient 8 was a 54-year-old (the oldest in the group) with predominantly frontal and parietal damage, but most of this damage was to the subcortical white matter. Klingman and Sussman (1983, p. 254) comment that:

> The fact that patient 8 ... had relatively spared cortex might speak to the importance of the integrity of underlying subcortical white matter (internal capsule specifically) in determining hemispheric capacity for language functions.

The patient had the best Boston Z score of the group and had suffered 2 CVAs six weeks apart some 7 years and 3 months earlier. This patient also produced the most marked evidence for right hemisphere mediation during both expressive and receptive tasks. The contrast between patients 1 and 8 is interesting because it illustrates the variability shown by the whole group in age (range 24 to 54 years), aetiology (gunshot wounds, road traffic accident, CVA), site and extent of lesion (frontal and anterior temporal, posterior inferior frontal and anterior temporal, posterior frontal, frontal, and parietal subcortical), as well as the variability in performance on the experimental tasks and Boston performance.

Further date are required from the interesting time-sharing technique. As the data stand they are difficult to interpret meaningfully and the possibility of lesion effects cannot be ignored; although the practice of establishing a pre-experimental tapping performance baseline, and determining degree of disruption by reference to this baseline, should control for possible lesion effects during the experimental condition. With reference to the essentially symmetrical disruption experienced by most of the aphasic group, Klingman and Sussman (1983) point out that:

> the time-sharing paradigm involving language presents such an enormous obstacle to the aphasic patient that interference is encountered regardless of tapping hand. this 'mass action' explanation, though not experimentally testable and not particularly enlightening, is nevertheless entirely plausible. It is offered as a precaution against overgeneralization from the lateralization data (p. 254).

Summary

So far we have examined the date which have accumulated over the years. They appear to suggest the participation of the right hemisphere in aphasia.

The evidence has come mainly from studies of patients who have suffered first left and then right hemisphere damage, and have demonstrated some degree of recovery between the two incidents only to become aphasic again following the second; from CT scan studies of patients who have sustained widespread left hemisphere damage but have shown significant recovery; from sodium amytal studies; and studies using various behavioural tests of hemispheric advantage or preference. Although there are grounds for accepting the general proposition for right hemisphere participation, there are problems of interpretation for much of the sodium amytal and behavioural evidence, especially where investigators have speculated too freely from often weak, circumstantial, and contaminated evidence.

Cases like those reported by Nielsen suggest that the right hemisphere may apparently take on responsibility for functions which have been lost or severely compromised in some individuals, while functions unaffected by the left hemisphere lesion are still processed by the left hemisphere. Interestingly, there appear to have been few of the bilateral lesion cases of the sort described by Neilsen reported in recent years. Why this should be so is unclear. The CT scan and some of the dichotic evidence points to a gradual, incremental involvement of the right hemisphere over time. CT scan, dichotic and sodium amytal data suggest that the right hemisphere is more likely to participate in patients with more severe aphasia (and probably more extensive left hemisphere damage) but less likely to be involved in milder cases.

Apart from the variability in quality of the evidence, a further major feature across studies is the apparent individual variability in patients. Both features conspire to mediate against the formulation of any general 'laws'. However, what does appear to be a relatively consistent finding across studies using different methodologies, is that right hemisphere participation may take place in patients who have severe aphasia, and that this involvement may increase with time. The evidence is not consistent, is not reliable, and has not been sufficiently replicated to allow us to go too far beyond this.

RIGHT HEMISPHERE INVOLVEMENT IN THE BEHAVIOURAL CHARACTERISTICS OF APHASIA

There have been few attempts to match the classic and familiar characteristics or features of aphasia with anything we know about, or can make reasonable guesses about, right hemisphere language. Most suggestions have been speculative with little supportive evidence. For instance, Brown (1981) reports that Niessl Von Mayendorff (1911) proposed that the jargonaphasia and paraphasia which sometimes follow a left temporal lobe lesion are the product of the inferior abilities of the corresponding area of the right hemisphere. Also, in Luria's opinion there is the possibility,

> of transfer of the disturbed function to the subordinate hemisphere and that it may be performed with the participation of the intact symmetrically opposite

zones of the subordinate hemisphere. The probability that the subordinate hemisphere may be involved in the peformance of functions (especially speech functions) hitherto effected by the dominant hemisphere is not constant but varies strongly from one subject to another (Luria, Naydin, Tsvetkova, and Vinarskaya, 1969, p. 379).

The kind of direct evidence necessary to examine detailed claims like these is simply not available. The investigations which have been carried out have been necessarily inferential, and the only symptoms which have received any significant attention are recurrent utterances and features of deep dyslexia. If it is the case, as discussion thus far suggests, that severely aphasic patients make some use of the right hemisphere, then this would indicate that some symptoms associated with severe aphasia may entail right hemisphere processing. It is interesting to note, therefore, that both recurrent utterances and deep dyslexia are associated with severe impairment and anterior damage.

In Chapter 5 it was suggested that the linguistic features of the recurrent utterances of severe Broca's aphasic patients seem to match up with what is known about right hemisphere processing capabilities. We will not go over the same ground at this point, but it was concluded that such factors as the non-propositionality of the expressions, their automatically and holistically produced nature, and their emotional character point to the involvement of the right hemisphere in their production. By far the most developed right hemisphere hypothesis has come about through work on the syndrome of deep dyslexia and we spend some time looking at this work below.

Deep dyslexia: the right hemisphere hypothesis

The rare collection of behavioural characteristics which make up the reading disorder first identified by Marshall and Newcombe (1973), and which has come to be known as deep dyslexia, is receiving increasing attention with regard to the possible contribution of the right hemisphere. Similarities exist between this disorder and the impairments of reading which accompany Broca's aphasia with agrammatism, but the 'pure' syndrome of deep dyslexia would appear to be relatively rare considering the number of individual cases which have been described (Coltheart, Patterson, and Marshall, 1980).

Reading aloud by patients with deep dyslexia is characterized by semantic errors (semantic paralexias), derivational errors like 'true' for 'truth' straight visual errors like 'shock' for 'stock', and an inability to read aloud invented words or non-words. There are particular problems with function words, which are either omitted or misread, and impairment in the ability to appreciate the phonological value of graphemes. This results in an inability to detect homophones—words which are pronounced the same but spelt differently—like 'maze' and 'maise' or 'night' and 'knight', and an inability to detect rhyming words which are spelt differently like 'fight' and 'kite'. The disorder is called 'deep dyslexia' because patients are thought to derive a direct semantic impression of a word without reference to its phonology

(Marshall and Newcombe, 1980; Coltheart, 1980a). The lesion in deep dyslexia is therefore one which severely impairs phonological processing in reading.

Coltheart (1980a) examined the linguistic capabilities of the right hemisphere and concluded that reading aloud in deep dyslexic patients was accomplished with significant right hemisphere participation. On Coltheart's right hemisphere model, deep dyslexia is due to a lesion which destroys the access between written orthography and the left hemisphere lexicon. Reading aloud, therefore, is accomplished by orthographic access to a right hemisphere lexicon and an interhemispheric transmission of semantic information to the left hemisphere. This information is then used to access an entry in the left hemisphere lexicon from which a phonological representation is retrieved and articulated by the left hemisphere.

The characteristic errors of deep dylexia can be accounted for by this route. Feature-loss semantic errors and function-word substitution errors, for instance, occur because the patient may tolerate a degree of difference between the semantic representation from the right hemisphere and the semantic representation in the left hemisphere lexicon. Associated semantic errors are due to incorrect selection of associated semantic words in the right hemisphere which are transmitted to the left hemisphere for production. Function-word omissions and substitutions occur because the right hemisphere is poor at processing syntax, hence there is difficulty in transmitting functors (which have little semantic representation) from the right to the left hemisphere (the model assumes that interhemispheric transmission of information is accomplished semantically). Semantic errors occur in abstract words because the right hemisphere is also poor at processing abstract words and is apt to produce errors; or, if the word has no semantic representation in the right hemisphere, interhemispheric transmission cannot take place. Alternatively, the word may be treated as a 'non-word' by the right hemisphere. Derivational errors may occur because the right hemisphere is simply unable to deal with inflectional forms. In summary, according to the model errors occur in reading aloud in deep dyslexic patients as a result of right hemisphere inadequacy and mismatch between right and left hemisphere representation.

Actual evidence for right hemisphere involvement in some of the features of reading, and also writing, in left-hemisphere-damaged patients comes from a handful of recent studies. A less detailed right hemiphere model of deep dyslexia has been proposed by Saffran, Bogyo, Schwartz, and Marin (1980). This model differs from Coltheart's in so far as it holds that most, if not all, processing takes place in the right hemisphere. The right hemisphere is responsible for the processing of all comprehension but actual encoding and production of speech may be performed by either hemisphere and may vary between patients. Saffran *et al.* present some experimental evidence in support of their hypothesis. Small groups of deep dyslexic subjects tested on a tachistoscopic lexical decision task and a dichotic digit task produced significantly superior left visual-field and left ear scores.

There are experimental findings which suggest that semantic paralexias are not restricted to deep dyslexic patients. Landis, Graves, and Goodglass (1982) produced evidence to suggest that the reading and writing of aphasic patients is significantly related to the emotional quality of words, and to the visual-field preferences of normal subjects. They tested the abilities of 8 fluent and 14 non-fluent aphasic patients to read aloud and write to dictation 12 abstract emotional words (e.g., 'fear', 'kill'), 12 concrete words (e.g., 'boat', 'lake'), and 12 abstract non-emotional words (e.g., 'time', 'view'). The generated data were compared to the tachistoscopic performance of 12 normal subjects (Graves, Landis, and Goodlass, 1981) using a mixture of the same sets of emotional and non-emotional words and pronounceable nonsense strings. Results showed that emotional words were read and written more accurately than both concrete and non-emotional abstract words by the aphasic subjects. In addition, significantly more paralexias and paragraphias were produced for emotional than for either concrete or non-emotional words. Moreover, it was also found that reading scores were highly correlated with normal left visual-field scores and not at all with normal right visual-field scores. Landis *et al*. conclude that:

> the present results raise the possibility that the language performances one frequently observes from aphasic patients indeed do reflect a substantial contribution from the undamaged hemisphere rather than just the remaining competence of the damaged, language dominant, hemisphere acting on its own (Landis *et al*., 1982, p. 110).

In a further study, Landis, Regard, Graves, and Goodglass (1983) examined relationships between lesion size and semantic paralexias in the same group of unselected aphasic patients. Analysis of the Landis *et al*. (1982) data had suggested that 11 out of 20 subjects had produced semantic paralexias. Of these 11, 9 had lesions which were almost triple the size of those without semantic paralexias as determined by CT scans. Interestingly, the presence of paralexia was not found to be significantly related to severity of aphasia. Possibly related to the finding that larger lesions correlate with semantic paralexias in aphasic patients, is Landis *et al*.'s (1983) observation that, in reading, it is those patients with smaller lesions and no semantic paralexias who apparently do not make use of the right hemisphere language system. In such patients, they suggest, a functional inhibition of the alternative right hemisphere system may be in operation.

Marshall and Patterson (1983) have challenged some of the findings from these studies. They firstly question whether many of the errors produced by the aphasic patients on reading and writing tasks are genuine *semantic* paralexias, suggesting instead that some could be seen as derivational and visual paralexias, or unrelated responses. However, there is no agreed definition of semantic error, and as the presence of such errors is meant to be the diagnostic cornerstone of deep dyslexia, the issue would appear to be an important one for future studies of reading in alexic and aphasic patients.

Secondly, Marshall and Patterson suggest that at least one of the subjects in the Landis *et al*. studies was probably a deep dyslexic. But the main concern of these writers is to question the operation of left hemisphere inhibition proposed by Landis *et al*. (1983), although, to be fair to Landis *et al*. they simply state that such inhibitory processes constitute *possible* explanations. Marshall and Patterson (1983) conclude:

> if the relevant zone of the right hemisphere produced only semantic errors in the normal brain, there would be obvious motivation for suppressing that area, but we assume that proponents of the right-hemisphere hypothesis believe that the relevant area would also produce *correct* responses when not inhibited. The patients in question read many words correctly, and we doubt that these authors would argue that the semantic errors arose in the right hemisphere but the correct responses in the left. If the right hemisphere can often process a printed word quite adequately to yield the correct oral response, would one not expect that two areas committed to the same function (albeit with differential efficiency) would co-operate with each other, rather than the stronger firmly inhibiting the contribution of the weaker side? (p. 426).

In a recent discussion, Coltheart (1983a) has attempted to address some of the challenges to the right hemisphere hypothesis of deep dyslexia. These have arisen from studies of pure alexia ('letter-by-letter reading') by Patterson and Kay (1982) and a newly described (in just one patient) *concrete-word dyslexia* by Warrington (1981). Typically, pure alexia arises from a lesion confined to the left occipital lobe and patients have little or no aphasia. Such patients should, therefore, have the right hemisphere reading system available to them and should be able to comprehend some written words, as deep dyslexics can. Patterson and Kay, however, found that such patients were unable to comprehend words unless they were able to read them aloud. The unique patient described by Warrington, in contrast to deep dyslexic patients, was better at reading abstract than concrete words. As discussed in several places in this book, the right hemisphere is thought to possess a better ability to process concrete words than abstract words. Therefore, why is it that patients with other forms of acquired alexia arising from unilateral left hemisphere lesions appear unable to access the right hemisphere reading system proposed to underlie the symptoms of deep dyslexia?

Coltheart (1983a) considers the possibility that some form of left hemisphere inhibition is operating in pure alexia and concrete-word dyslexia to prevent access to the right hemisphere. The concrete-word dyslexic described by Warrington was examined within 20 days of onset, and the evidence discussed so far in this chapter indicates that right hemisphere involvement in language following left hemisphere damage may take some time to emerge. For the deep dyslexic patients who have been described, on the other hand, the required symptoms have not emerged for at least one year after brain damage. Coltheart, therefore, raises the possibility that the patient described by Warrington would not have shown evidence of right hemisphere reading so soon post-onset. Pure alexic patients typically read in a letter-by-letter fashion, have little or no aphasic impairment, a right homonymous hemianopia and small lesions restricted to the left occipital lobe, often including the splenium of the corpus callosum. Given the evidence discussed earlier, which suggests that right hemisphere linguistic competence may only emerge following substantial damage to the left hemisphere, pure alexic patients may be unable to access the right hemisphere because the relatively intact left hemisphere suppresses the right's reading system.

However, Coltheart (1983a) points out with regard to concrete-word dyslexia:

> this kind of explanation cannot be offered if one at the same time wishes to argue that normal readers (in whom this suppression, of course, ought to be at its strongest) exhibit evidence of right hemisphere contributions to the reading of concrete words (p. 190).

For C.A.V., the concrete-word dyslexic reported by Warrington, Coltheart (1983a) prefers instead an alternative analysis of the results of the study which appears to demonstrate that 'it is far from obvious that one can claim that the more concrete a word the less likely it was that C.A.V. could read it correctly ... it seems fair to conclude that a clearer demonstration of concrete-word dyslexia is needed before one need regard the existence of this disorder as a decisive refutation of the view that the right hemisphere possesses some reading capability' (pp. 188–189).

Coltheart proposes that for pure alexia there is an impairment in interhemispheric transfer of information from right to left hemisphere which produces the slow characteristic letter-by-letter reading. He argues that the poor performance by the right hemisphere in the normal reader on abstract words, non-words, and *kana* is because the right hemisphere cannot categorize these stimuli semantically. Semantically categorized information cannot therefore be transferred to the left for decision making. (The left hemisphere is fully responsible still for all expressive processing on Coltheart's model.) The normal right hemisphere can categorize these stimuli orthographically and sends the results of this to the left hemisphere as well as uncategorized information. The normal reader, therefore, uses categorized and uncategorized interhemispheric transfer. The left hemisphere of the deep dyslexic, on the other hand, cannot identify orthographical information but the right can perform semantic categorization. The result of this categorization—a semantic representation—is transferred to the left. Finally, the letter-by-letter reading of the pure alexic is because the left hemisphere—deprived of direct input from the right visual-field by the right homonymous hemianopia—receives either uncategorized letter representations from the right hemisphere or categorized but degraded information due to a second lesion, probably to the splenium of the corpus callosum.

The debate on right brain involvement in deep dyslexia continues with a recent review by Patterson and Besner (1984) with commentaries by

Rabinowicz and Moscovitch (1984) and Zaidel and Schweiger (1984). In their comprehensive critique Patterson and Besner detail a number of important problems for the right hemisphere hypothesis. They firstly question the quality of much of Coltheart's source evidence: the equivocal nature of most of the available data together with the total lack of respectable levels of replication.

Patterson and Besner also provide data which seriously undermine Coltheart's proposal that deep dyslexic reading corresponds closely with the reading competence of the separated right hemisphere. Their comparison of the written word and sentence comprehension of two deep dyslexic patients with Zaidel's (1978a, 1982) results for split-brain subjects N.G. and L.B. showed that the deep dyslexics were far superior to the separated right hemisphere on reading subtests of the Boston and Western Aphasia Tests and the Peabody Picture Vocabulary Test. This means, they suggest, that either the right hemispheres of N.G. and L.B. have poorer language skills than the normal right hemisphere or that reading performance by deep dyslexic patients reflects more than right hemisphere reading. While accepting that 'the correspondence between deep dyslexic and RH reading is at best one of partial identity' (p. 353), Zaidel and Schweiger (1984) point out that the differences could be due to greater variability between individuals in right hemisphere language competence and the size of the right hemisphere lexicon. Moreover, the right hemisphere role in any aspect of linguistic processing may not necessarily be a fixed and pre-determined one; it may act more like a back-up system helping out when the left hemisphere is overloaded or tired.

Summary

We have looked in detail at the important work on deep dyslexia in this chapter, and at recurrent utterances in Chapter 4. It is only in recent years that more systematic investigation has been directed towards the question of whether the right hemisphere is to any extent responsible for neural control during processing of the characteristics of aphasia. For recurrent utterances, it was concluded that the presence or absence of particular features of their linguistic structure, and the available evidence on the involvement of the right hemisphere in speech production, provides support for the view that at least the real-word type could be produced by the right hemisphere. Similarly, it has been argued, there is more than a coincidental relationship between the features of deep dyslexia and what is known of right hemisphere language.

A general weakness in the argument is that the approach for these investigations has been essentially inferential: investigators have attempted to match-up current knowledge on what the right hemisphere can achieve with the symptoms observed in aphasic patients. Clearly this inferential approach is not ideal; we do not have a stable knowledge base for right hemisphere language. We can therefore expect developments in our understanding of right hemisphere language to modify inferences about the activity of the right hemisphere in aphasic language. In addition, physiological investigations are required to examine such hypotheses more fully.

Do the discussions on deep dyslexia and other forms of alexia provide any grounds for considering a significant right hemisphere involvement in other features of language disorder following left hemisphere damage? To what extent can we entertain the idea that some or all of the actual behavioural characteristics of aphasia which we observe are the products of the right hemisphere? Apart from the work already discussed there has been little direct study of this question. however, the level of understanding that we now have of right hemisphere language allows us at least to suggest that some options are more likely than others.

The option that *all* aphasic behavioural characteristics represent just right hemisphere activity is highly unlikely. Our fuller appreciation of the importance of individual differences, for instance, as well as a more detailed appreciation of the complexity of aphasia (both discussed in Chapter 2) suggest instead, that if there is right hemisphere involvement in aphasic symptomatology then it is at a much more differentiated and selective level. In the absence of good evidence we cannot take speculation too far. None the less, the arguments made in favour of right hemisphere involvement in deep dyslexia might also be applied to other aspects of language impairment in brain damage. It can be noted that such features as semantic errors (semantic or verbal paraphasia), observable in a range of aphasia types, difficulty with function words in agrammatism, and a tendency towards success with words which are concrete, high in frequency and imagery on naming tasks, are not only features of deep dyslexia. In addition there is the finding already discussed at some length that emotionality is also a characteristic of aphasic language, and this may implicate the right hemisphere.

There is a rich area here for future research. Recent years have seen the development of a much more systematic approach to research in neuropsychology. Our confidence in the reliability of future research findings should therefore increase.

CONCLUSIONS: THE APHASIC RIGHT HEMISPHERE?

Our discussion has shown that there is a small range of physiological and behavioural evidence—not all of which stands up to close scrutiny—which generally supports the lateral shift hypothesis. Early on we suggested that there appeared really to be several major alternatives of the hypothesis, each asking different questions. Our examination has found that an increased research effort in recent years has helped to state these questions more clearly for future studies, and a number of areas would appear to make promising candidates for more intensive attention.

It appears as if the view that the right hemisphere takes over in some blanket fashion in most aphasic patients is unlikely. From the evidence available, the indications are that not all aphasic patients make a shift to the right. Is it the case that the right hemisphere takes over incrementally? That is to say, if the left loses, say, 10% of its language function because of damage, does that mean that the right makes up the difference in some sense? A 30% loss of function in the left would produce a corresponding 30% increase in language activity in the right, and so on. The first objection to such an idea is that the right is not able to offer a fully equivalent back-up system. The right hemisphere substitution is always going to be inferior to the lost left hemisphere function. In addition, the evidence presented throughout this text suggests that the right hemisphere's contribution will not be the same as the left's, nor simply less. Methods which have been used are perhaps still a little too crude to tease out the kind of detailed information necessary to investigate seriously such an unlikely possibility. If the right hemisphere is significantly involved in recovery from aphasia, then its role would appear to be a more complex and differentiated one. A range of sources suggest that its involvement is related to severity of aphasic impairment and time since onset of left hemisphere damage.

A further possibility is that different aphasia types have separate hemispheric involvement. That is to say, certain *syndromes* may be made up of symptoms processed predominantly by the right hemisphere, as has been claimed for deep dyslexia. Such syndromes would appear to be those most associated with severe aphasic impairment of long standing, as is the case with deep dyslexia. If this were the case it would suggest that such right hemisphere syndromes only emerge in the presence of major left hemisphere insult that fails to recover. It is conceivable at least, that some aphasia types represent essentially right hemisphere processing. Thus the symptom complex which makes up what is conventionally recognized as a particular and independent type of aphasia would need to be processed entirely by the right hemisphere. Although severity appears to be a relevant factor, it would seem inappropriate to interpret this finding to support the position that *global* aphasia here represents an aphasia type in the generally accepted sense. Apart from the question of whether classification of patients into taxonomic types is a useful strategy for research (Caramazza, 1984), the term global is used mainly descriptively for patients who have severe deficits in all modalities, rather than as a theoretically independent type of aphasia. The available evidence does not allow an investigation of what, given the complexity of aphasic symptomatology, must also be an unlikely possibility.

A further more differentiated possibility, is that certain behavioural characteristics of aphasia are processed by the right hemisphere. So, it may be the case that certain symptoms represent significant right hemisphere involvement in most individual cases, as was suggested for real-word recurrent utterances and some features of deep dyslexia in the last section. Again, it may be those symptoms, like recurrent utterances and deep dyslexia, which are associated with severe aphasia of long standing. The evidence discussed in this chapter provides some support for this more differentiated view, but firm conclusion would be premature and inappropriate at this stage in our understanding, especially in the absence of hard physiological evidence. What recent research has produced, however, is firstly, a deeper appreciation that right hemisphere involvement in language processing following left hemisphere damage is probably dependent upon a complex interplay of a range of variables, and secondly, a clearer picture of the range of testable questions which make up the lateral shift hypothesis.

Most recent progress has come about through the comprehensive investigation of aphasic patients using intensive single case methodology. As more carefully designed studies are conducted, and improved physiological techniques increase our confidence in findings, our understanding of the underlying neurophysiological and information-processing mechanisms involved in right hemisphere processing following left hemisphere damage should only be enriched.

Chapter Eight

THE ROLE OF THE RIGHT HEMISPHERE IN THE REHABILITATION OF APHASIA

The purpose of this chapter is to examine the clinical implications of right hemisphere involvement in communication. We will be concerned with the possible and potential role of the right hemisphere in the rehabilitation of aphasia.

Approaches to the rehabilitation of aphasia exist which are based, either by design or accident, on surviving right hemisphere modes of processing information. For the most part these methods are reorganizational approaches which aim to replace the lost function with another compensatory function, as opposed to re-establishing impaired or lost functions. The terms re-establishment and reorganizational, as used by Rosner (1970), are not mutually exclusive and are employed quite loosely and generally in rehabilitation. Thus, Melodic Intonation Therapy, which will be discussed more fully later, aims to re-establish speech in aphasic patients, as far as is possible, by reorganization of the process of speech production using melodic intonation. In this use of the terms a right hemisphere function (melodic intonation) is used to aid a left hemisphere function (segmental speech production) through a reorganizational process. Below we examine some examples of rehabilitation methods which may either compensate using right hemisphere functions or re-establish lost functions through some form of neurocognitive reorganization involving the right hemisphere. Following this discussion of already more or less established methods, we examine some more recently suggested approaches based on improvements in our understanding of right hemisphere functioning.

COMPENSATION UTILIZING RIGHT HEMISPHERE FUNCTION

The most obvious methods which appear to utilize right hemisphere cognitive functions are those which employ artificial languages made up of visual arbitrary shapes, or ideographic and iconographic symbols and signs. the pioneering work in this area was a study by Glass, Gazzaniga, and Premack (1973) with subsequent work by Gardner and associates (Baker, Berry, Gardner, Zurif, Davis, and Veroff, 1975; Gardner, Zurif, Berry, and Baker, 1976) and a more clinically orientated application by Carrier (1974) and Carrier and Peck (1974).

The Glass *et al.* study employed a modification of the coloured arbitrary shapes system used by Premack (1971) to assess the abilities of chimpanzees to acquire and use an artificial language. These shapes are functionally equivalent to words and employ left-to-right sequencing. Seven global aphasic patients with minimal residual language and no apparent syntactic competence were selected to be taught the system. Despite very severe aphasia the patients were described as alert, bright-eyed and well motivated, with substantial non-verbal abilities. Patients were given varying amounts of training which initially entailed arranging a mixture of symbols and 'words' (e.g., two objects with the symbol for 'same' or 'different' between them). 'Sentences' or strings were gradually built up until the patients could manage to ask a question like 'Anthea (experimenter's name) give John (patient's name) water' (p. 98). Patients were taught a vocabulary of nouns and verbs as well as the use of symbols for interrogation and negation. Patients were able to achieve a level of skill with this language far beyond their abilities with natural language.

Gardner *et al.* (1976) called the system they developed VIC (visual communication). It consisted of a range of arbitrary (geometric) or representational (ideographic) symbols drawn individually on small cards. Unlike the Glass *et al.* system, therefore, some symbols were actually schematic object pictures (e.g., the object 'glass' was denoted by a drawing of a glass tumbler and 'to go home' was a drawing of a car arriving at the front of a house). Training was conducted at two levels. Level 1 entailed carrying out commands—where the patient was given an instruction using the cards (e.g., pick up an object), answering questions, and describing events. Successful patients then went on to Level 2 which explored the ability to express needs, feelings, and desires using the system. VIC, like the Glass *et al.* system, used a left-to-right syntax with the agent of the action appearing at the beginning of the 'sentence'. Symbol types included nouns, verbs, prepositions, conjunctions, a range of *wh* symbols, adjectives as well as message category markers to distinguish between interrogative, declarative, and emphatic forms which were functionally equivalent to question and answer and exclamation marks. This study also chose severe global aphasic patients, most of whom were at least six months post-onset, who had made minimal progress with more conventional therapy and who were able to match objects to pictures.

Both these studies reported remarkable success, with global patients being able to learn the systems and use them in the clinics for what must be considered propositional communication. Moreover, patients were seen to be far superior in their abilities to use these artificial systems than they were with natural language. The relative success of these similar systems with globally aphasic patients raises some interesting questions. Firstly, it provides support for the view that linguistic competence is preserved following left hemisphere damage and that it is linguistic performance which is impaired, as is proposed by Weigl and Bierwisch (1970). The globally aphasic patients in these studies were not simply matching shapes to objects, but were creating new and original sentences by arranging and rearranging 'words'—i.e., they were using a syntactic code. The interesting question is, was it the right hemisphere which was learning the new system and adapting its visuospatial and predominantly holistic abilities to a linear sequencial task? This would suggest that even globally aphasic individuals retain some form of syntactic ability. Gazzaniga (1974b) suggests in his discussion of this work that:

> the implicit functional syntactic mechanism present and active in decoding a meaningful array is probably able to come to the assistance of the organism when the syntactic mechanism for language has been destroyed through stroke or lesion (p. 205).

A further important property that these systems possess which makes them different from natural spoken language is their quasi-permanent nature. The message is laid in front of the patient who has ample time to process and manipulate information. Sufficient time would therefore be available for a right hemisphere Gestalt cognitive mode to take in the 'sentence' and decode the holistic message in the same way that it decodes any pictorial array. As Horner and Fedor (1983) point out, with these systems the characteristic auditory processing deficit in aphasia is bypassed and their quasi-permanent nature means that the memory load is far less than with temporally organized auditory stimuli.

What may also be of significance from these studies and others which have attempted to teach aphasic patients alternative methods of communication, including the use of electronic communication aids (DiSimoni, 1981; Enderby and Hamilton, 1983), is that patients appear to demonstrate a high degree of 'comsumer resistance' to artificial methods and devices. This resistance is probably much higher among aphasic than other groups (for instance, severely anarthric or laryngectomy patients), who usually welcome any alternative system that enhances communicative effectiveness. It appears that some aphasic individuals may have difficulty in accepting artificial languages, gestural systems, and communication aids as genuine alternatives to conventional oral–aural speech outside the clinical situation. Gardner *et al.* make the point that patients may simply view such systems as elaborate 'games' and not related to real communication at all. This may simply be a reflection of their unwillingness to accept that speech will never return, but it may also be the case that there are other—cognitive—factors involved which may prevent left-hemisphere-damaged patients from recognizing a potentially useful system which can help with communication.

Other visually based systems which have been used with aphasic patients are Non-Slip (None Speech Language Initiation Program) developed from the work reviewed above (Carrier, 1974; Carrier and Peak, 1974) and the Blissymbolics system (Saya, 1979; Bailey, 1983). The Non-Slip system is commercially available and includes various sizes of arbitrary geometric coloured shapes, each with the word it represents printed on it, and picture cards used as stimuli for sentence construction. The Blissymbolics system includes a lexicon of 100 mixed symbols and signs, including numerals, mathematical symbols, punctuation signs and a range of arbitrary geometric, ideographic and iconographic forms. The word or phrase that the symbol or sign represents is also printed alongside on a communication board. Varying degrees of success have been reported with these approaches to rehabilitation. Interestingly, Bailey conducted a *post hoc* tachistoscopic investigation of her single patient which revealed a left visual-field advantage for verbal material. However, it is not possible to determine whether the Bliss programme *per se* was responsible for this left visual-field advantage.

Right hemisphere imagery and rehabilitation

Assuming the validity of the theory that different cognitive modes are associated with the two hemispheres of the brain then aphasic patients will be more impaired in their abilities to perform analytic and serial tasks associated with the left hemisphere functional mode than holistic and synthetic tasks associated with right hemisphere processing. It might therefore make sense to develop and explore therapeutic approaches which appear to entail holistic/ Gestalt rather than analytic/serial processing.

There has been developing in aphasia therapy a shift away from a rigid clinical and linguistic emphasis in assessment and treatment towards a more functional and pragmatic approach (e.g., Prutting, 1982; Davis and Wilcox, 1985). This can be seen in the emergence and increasing popularity of 'functional' assessment procedures like the Functional Communication Profile (Taylor-Sarno, 1969), the Communicative Abilities in Daily Living evaluation (Holland, 1980). Such procedures are concerned not with assessing a patient's level of ability with strict linguistic skills, but in determining the patient's level of communicative competence. In parallel with these developments is the increased emphasis on more functionally and naturalistically appropriate approaches to treatment such as the 'PACE' (Promoting Aphasics Communicative Effectiveness) method (Davis and Wilcox, 1981, 1985) and 'VAT' (Visual Action Therapy) method (Helm-Easterbrook, Fitzpatrick and Barresi, 1982).

West (1983) has suggested that an approach to therapy could be:

> to use naturalistic, conversational settings that are highly redundant and have rich contexts so that the patient is able to extract as much as possible from the nonlinguistic context itself (p. 217).

The PACE method adopts essentially this approach. On the face of it, such a naturalistic communicative process involves a global, holistic appreciation of the pragmatic context of the message on the part of the aphasic communicator and places minimal emphasis on analytic and sequential skills. It is just those features of communication, such as facial expression, prosody and pragmatics, which the preceding discussion has indicated are mediated by the right hemisphere.

West (1983) has proposed a theoretical rationale for a form of therapy for aphasia based on heightening visual imagery. She reviews the research on imagery, concreteness and meaningfulness of words, which has demonstrated that normal subjects perform better on a variety of learning and memory tasks with words which are high in imagery and concreteness than on words which are low in imagery and concreteness. As discussed in some detail in Chapter 2 of this volume, findings from this area of research provide grounds to believe that language is mediated via the two coding systems of verbal symbolism and non-verbal visual imagery. These two systems are seen as functioning either independently or in cooperation through the action of the left (verbal symbolic) and right (visual imagery) hemispheres. If the functioning of the verbal code is impaired through left hemisphere damage, then, as West points out, this does not necessarily mean that the right hemisphere's contribution to linguistic processing via visual imagery is unavailable:

if one uses concrete pictures as treatment stimuli, then both the verbal and imagery code may be aroused. In aphasics, the capacity to arouse the verbal code is depressed, if not absent, but these stimuli still hold the potential to arouse the visual code, which is presumably unimpaired. Furthermore, if one code is able to assist in indirectly arousing the other, then arousal of the visual code may in some cases facilitate arousal of the verbal code (p. 226).

As West (1983) points out, a number of studies have shown that aphasic subjects perform better on tasks when encouraged to use visual imagery. Edelstein (1976) found that aphasic subjects perform better on a recognition memory task for words when provided with a description of the word designed to heighten visual imagery, plus a picture to accompany the word. Cannezzio (1977) found, not surprisingly, that aphasic subjects produced faster reaction times in a word-matching task with high as opposed to low imagery words.

In addition, it has been proposed that action words, or words which are 'operative' (Gardner, 1973; West, 1978) are processed better by the right hemisphere. Myers (1980, p. 69) has suggested that an image is not simply a static picture but a dynamic,

nonverbal confluence of emotion, intellect and sensation. It is a simultaneous integration of multiple levels of perceived (or interpreted) experience which contains the intersection of many currents of feeling and thought. It thereby violates any one-to-one or type-token correspondence with real objects or events.

Myers goes on to suggest that the use of stimulus materials aimed at encouraging imagery in the treatment of aphasia, should therefore involve highly imageable actions which entail complex relationships and interactions. Such images are stronger, she proposes, perhaps because relationships are suggested which require interpretation and invoke rich associations.

West and Myers are arguing that not only should linguistic stimuli chosen for use in treatment sessions be high in imagery, concreteness, meaningfulness, and rich contextual associations, but that programmes should be designed, and evaluated, which encourage patients to use visual imagery and maximize what appears to be an intact cognitive strategy mediated by the undamaged right hemisphere.

RE-ESTABLISHMENT VIA RIGHT HEMISPHERE REORGANIZATION

A further class of therapeutic methods in use which probably utilize right hemisphere functional abilities ars those which, unlike the artificial systems described in the preceding section, aim to re-establish speech. These methods are Melodic Intonation Therapy (MIT) developed by Sparks and co-workers (Albert, Sparks, and Helm, 1973; Sparks, Helm, and Albert, 1974; Sparks, 1981) and the 'preventive method' reported by Beyn and Shokher-Trotskaya (1966).

Melodic Intonation Therapy is deliberately based on the research discussed in Chapter 5 that indicates that the right hemisphere has special responsibilities for the processing of music and prosody and severe Broca's patients often retain remarkable abilities to sing and use prosodic features. This is thought to underlie the ability to pronounce the words of songs with a skill that is far in excess of the ability to pronounce the same words in a non-musical context. The method involved a strict behavioural training programme where patients learn to produce two- to four-word utterances using a simple, but musically exaggerated intonation contour.

The 'preventive' method described by Beyn and Shokher-Trotskaya does not claim to have anything to do with involvement of the right hemisphere, but the right hemisphere may contribute to its reported success. The method is aimed at preventing the emergence of agrammatism in Broca's patients by discouraging the use of object naming and complex propositional speech in the first few weeks post-onset of the aphasia. Patients are encouraged instead to use single words (not nouns) expressing a whole idea ('predicates') in combination with exaggerated and varying intonation patterns like, 'Oh!', 'No!', 'There!', 'Here!', 'Give!', 'Take!', etc. Auxiliary and modal verbs (e.g., 'shall', 'will', 'can') and pronouns and adverbs are gradually introduced later. The emergence of agrammatism was reported to have been prevented in 25 patients who would have been reasonably expected to have developed it. Patients were able to move from these restricted utterances to non-agrammatic speech, and when spontaneous words began to emerge at two to six weeks, general nouns were introduced, but not object nouns.

The authors suggest that what this approach to the problem of agrammatism does is to avoid the 'nominative system' of speech which is what becomes 'fixed' in agrammatic speech. The prevention of agrammatism in these patients using this method could be due to an early use and stimulation of right hemisphere forms of language, although this was not the authors' interpretation for the reported success of the method. The use of single holistic utterances, modal verbs, emotional–reactive speech and exaggerated intonation, with a parallel inhibition of attempts at nominative and segmental utterances, could mean that damaged left hemisphere mechanisms, which may be responsible for agrammatism, are bypassed. What is of further interest is that since the original report of this work, no replication studies of the preventive method have been reported and the method does not appear to have been widely applied.

Hypnosis, aphasia, and the right hemisphere

There are some interesting indications that a possible future approach to aphasia rehabilitation involving right hemisphere processing might be developed from some recent studies which have examined the relationship between hypnosis and hemispheric processing (Gur and Gur, 1974; Frumkin, Ripley, and Cox, 1978; McKeever, Larrabee, Sullivan, Johnson, Ferguson, and Rayport, 1981). Gur and Gur found significant interactions between lateral eye movements during verbal and spatial questioning in 60 right-handed male and female subjects while under hypnosis; although handedness, sex, and eyedness were found to be moderating variables. The results are interpreted to suggest that the right hemisphere has a special involvement during hypnosis. Frumkin *et al.* tested 10 male and 10 female subjects on a dichotic CVC syllable test before hypnosis, during hypnosis, and following hypnosis. Significantly reduced right ear scores were observed during hyp-nosis suggesting to the investigators that the right hemisphere is markedly more affected by hypnotic trance than the left.

While no specific treatment approach to aphasia has been developed incorporating hypnosis, these recent suggestions that the right hemisphere is affected to a greater extent by hypnosis than the left hemisphere might provide a basis for an approach to treatment. Such an idea gains some impetus from a recent study which examined the effects of right hemisphere hypnosis on a commissurotomized patient (McKeever *et al.*, 1981). In this study a 28-year-old female split-brain patient was tested for left hand tactile anomia before, during, and following hypnotic trance. As discussed in Chapter 3 such individuals are markedly deficient in their ability to name objects which are palpated by the left hand, due to the disconnection between the left hand tactile input and the left hemisphere caused by the sectioning of the corpus callosum. During the non-hypnotic pre-test the subject named 2 out of 20 objects palpated with the left hand. During hypnosis, 7 days later, the experimenters were concerned to have the subject regress to childhood in the hope that this strategy might result in more right hemisphere speech. The patient was a good subject and apparently regressed back to age 11 years. When asked to write her name with her left hand (right hemisphere), she wrote her maiden name and was also able to write her teacher's name. In addition, she was able to name 7 out of 21 objects presented to the left hand (right hemisphere). Her speech was reported to be slow and extremely effortful. Following hypnosis the subject was tested again and could name only one item.

During a second hypnotic session when the subject was apparently not in as deep a trance as the first session, she was able to name 5 items from 21 under age regression, and just 3 from 21 without regression. However, during a third session, when the subject was clearly in a deep trance, she named 11 out of 21 objects; but, surprisingly, following a 10-minute break, was able to name 12 out of 21 without hypnosis. The authors suggest that this high score was due to the probability that the subject simply fell back into the hypnotic state when she returned to the same room and the same comfortable chair. A subsequent session produced a low score without hypnosis (2 out of 21) and a high score (11 out of 21) under hypnosis.

The authors suggest that improvements in naming under hypnosis might simply be due to a relaxed state or, possibly, the suppression of guessing by the left hemisphere, which, they conjecture, may be responsible for poor guessing without hypnosis. They also speculate that the laboured speech observed could be a result of right hemisphere control of left hemisphere speech production mechanisms via the patient's intact anterior commissure.

On the face of it there would appear to be a basis here for a series of studies to examine the possible role of hypnosis, or even deep relaxation, in aphasia therapy. A number of intriguing questions arise from McKeever *et al.*'s (1981) study for future studies: What might the relationship be between the slow laboured speech observed in this subject and the slow laboured speech of Broca's aphasic patients? Could this speech have been the product of the right hemisphere? With verbally impaired aphasic patients will hypnotic induction be more difficult, or is it the case that induction is more dependent on the prosodic aspects of speech for success? With successful induction in an aphasic patient, what might be the expected effects on the relationship between a hypnotized damaged left hemisphere and a hypnotized intact right hemisphere, i.e., might the hypothesized effects of left hemisphere inhibition of right hemisphere language capacities be reduced?

Although the results of studies with artificial languages are of immense theoretical and practical interest, and of potential value with globally affected patients, the methods which utilize oral–aural approaches are clearly ones which would be preferred by patients who are capable of achieving the necessary levels of ability to commence such programmes. Aphasic patients want to use speech. They do not appear to be impressed, for whatever reason, by cards, shapes and gestures, but what has always been the most efficient and natural mode of communication. More success in terms of transfer to non-clinical situations and generalization to natural communication situations may therefore occur with methods which attempt to re-establish via reorganization rather than compensate via reorganization.

Horner and Fedor (1983) have recently brought together many of the findings on hemispheric processing, the assumptions of the holistic–analytic theory, the concept of deblocking, and the ideas and results of studies so far detailed in this chapter to outline an approach to the treatment of aphasia which includes the idea of hemisphere reorganization. The approach advocated by Horner and Fedor essentially claims to achieve access to impaired processes associated with damaged Broca's or Wernicke's areas in the left hemisphere, via the right hemisphere's homologous 'Broca's' and 'Wernicke's' areas and their connecting fasciculi and transcallosal pathways. The tasks employed in therapy are selected to achieve the goal of facilitating or deblocking the impaired function.

Horner and Fedor present some fairly detailed tables of how treatment for impaired expression and comprehension in Broca's and Wernicke's aphasic patients might proceed utilizing intact right hemisphere functions. For instance, the suggested treatment of agrammatism focuses on the linguistic levels of prosody, phonology and syntax, with targets arranged in a hierarchy of difficulty within each level. At each level of treatment 'deblockers' are paired. This involves the pairing of an intact function—assumed to be processed by the undamaged right hemisphere—and an impaired function. For example, the initial aim at the prosodic level is to re-establish control of volitional phonation. This, it is suggested, may be achieved by pairing prosodic–affective deblockers (e.g., emotional facial expression) and visual–spatial–holistic deblockers (e.g., whole body movements) with vocalization. The interesting and comprehensive programme proposed by Horner and Fedor is based on a fairly uncritical acceptance of the findings reported in the literature and is as yet clinically untested.

RE-ESTABLISHMENT VIA HEMISPHERIC SPECIALIZATION RETRAINING

The approaches and suggested approaches to aphasia rehabilitation so far considered aim to some degree or other to utilize the apparent natural abilities of the right hemisphere. In this section we examine the few single-case studies which have explored the possibilities of re-establishing linguistic skills in aphasic patients via a more direct attempt actually to reorganize cognitive processing in the right hemisphere. Given that the evidence surveyed in earlier chapters (particularly in Chapter 6) supports the view that the right hemisphere is not simply capable of compensating for lost left hemisphere functions, but is also able to adapt in such a way that it is capable of subserving left hemisphere type linguistic processes, then an approach to rehabilitation which aims to stimulate a pre-existing but latent right hemisphere linguistic capability, or actually teach the right hemisphere new skills— left hemisphere skills—would certainly appear to be worth investigation.

The first problem, however, is deciding what the objectives of a 'hemispheric specialization retaining' (HSR) programme might be and what effects it might conceivably have. A broad objective might be to re-establish some lost linguistic skill following left hemisphere damage. The programme might hope to achieve this objective either through stimulation of available but latent right hemisphere linguistic abilities or by causing new learning to take place in the right hemisphere. There is neurophysiological evidence which suggests that general stimulation is capable of promoting behavioural recovery following brain damage in animals and that this recovery coincides with neurochemical changes in brain tissue (John, 1982). If the view is taken that the right hemisphere is unlikely to possess sufficient latent linguistic ability to effect any major improvements in function, then a programme which aims actually to cause new learning to take place might stand a better chance of success. This might mean that the right hemisphere would need to start from scratch to acquire, through learning, the necessary skills to process the kinds of linguistic material for which it is not naturally specialized.

Differentiation between these two explanations for observed improvement following an HSR programme would not be easy. It may be achieved by noting the rate of improvement in abilities and comparisons of pre- and post-treatment measures of hemispheric preference for verbal material. A large and once-and-for-all improvement in abilities correlated with a similar large increase in left lateral preference scores could indicate a wholesale linguistic competence shift hypothesis. A gradual improvement in communicative abilities coupled with a progressive increase in left lateral preference would tend to support a right hemisphere learning hypothesis. The former might suggest that the programme had acted to trigger or release latent right hemisphere linguistic skills, freeing them from some form of left hemisphere inhibition.

Prima facie, it would appear that a right hemisphere learning hypothesis is asking a great deal of a mature right hemisphere. It seems unlikely, however, that the right hemisphere would actually have to 'learn language' from scratch and therefore take the same sort of time scale as a developing child, as has been suggested (Powell, 1981). Firstly, the research indicates that the right hemisphere can no longer be considered entirely devoid of language skills, but plays a significant role even in 'linguistic' processing. Secondly, an 'average' aphasic patient, although having deficits in specific areas, also has substantial retained abilities. Having selected a subject with certain specific linguistic deficits, the aim of an HSR programme would be to provide training in those skills which appear to underlie the specific deficit areas, not to 'reteach' an entire human language.

Even so, this is not to underestimate what is being asked of the right hemisphere. An HSR programme would require the right hemisphere to learn a mode of processing for which the available evidence suggests it is by nature unsuited and may even be the sole domain of the left hemisphere in the normal right-handed individual. It is not simply requiring the right hemisphere to use its own specialized functions in a compensatory way, but is asking a mature right hemisphere to learn a sequential, segmental, temporal mode of processing, because this is the mode of processing which appears to underlie the linguistic processing capabilities of the left hemisphere, and these are the functions which appear to be impaired following left hemisphere damage.

Just two studies have been reported which have attempted to investigate the possibility of improving the linguistic abilities of aphasic subjects by directly stimulating the right hemisphere (Buffery and Burton, 1982; Code, 1983). Both studies independently selected a relatively young, male subject with Wernicke's aphasia secondary to a CVA and of similar time since onset. Both studies utilized tachistoscopic viewing, dichotic listening, and haptic manipulation. (See Chapter 2 for critical evaluation of these techniques.) Moore (1974) and Buffery (1977) had suggested that methods were available for directing treatment materials to a specific hemisphere and that programmes could be designed around these methods. Buffery called his approach 'brain function therapy' (Buffery, 1977; Buffery and Burton, 1982), and it should be noted that his conception of brain function therapy (BFT) differs quite markedly from the more general use of the term by Powell (1981), who describes BFT in terms of a general cognitive and behavioural approach to the rehabilitation of brain damaged patients.

The essence of the BFT method is illustrated by Figure 6 (from Buffery and Burton, 1982). The subject of Buffery's study was a Wernicke's aphasic patient in his 'late forties' who had sustained a series of left hemisphere strokes. Treatment began some two years after his last CVA and he was assumed to be beyond any period of natural or spontaneous recovery. The subject had a slight right-sided hemiparesis, a mild right visual-field defect, and a severe aphasia. Treatment first worked through the visual, auditory, and tactile modalities separately and progressed to a cross-tri-modal condition using all three modalities. Tasks progressed from the simple to the more complex. In the tachistoscopic condition, for instance, single letters progressed to words and material was presented to the LVF with digits at fixation. The dichotic condition presented verbal material to the left ear while presenting 'neutral' white noise to the right ear. Similarly, in the haptic condition, verbal material was presented to the left hand and a neutral sponge to the right. The programme worked up to a cross-tri-modal semantic discrimination task. In the example shown in Figure 6 the subject's task was to identify 'toy' as the odd one out.

The subject's ongoing progress with treatment tasks was periodically sampled to determine whether improvement was taking place. This showed a gradual increase in left lateral responses over the treatment period (approximately 2 years, 6 months). In addition, the Wechsler Adult Intelligence Scale and Wechsler–Bellvue Intelligence Scales were periodically administered. Most interestingly, Verbal IQ improved from a level at initial assessment where testing was not possible, gradually increasing to an average 101 by the end of treatment. Furthermore, there was no reduction in scores on performance tests during the period, which the authors took to indicate that improvement in verbal skills by the right hemisphere was not at the expense of spatial–holistic processing.

J.W., the subject of Code's (1983c) HSR study, was a 37-year-old right-handed male Wernicke's aphasic who had suffered a thromboembolic CVA some four years before the study commenced. CT scan and EEG confirmed a

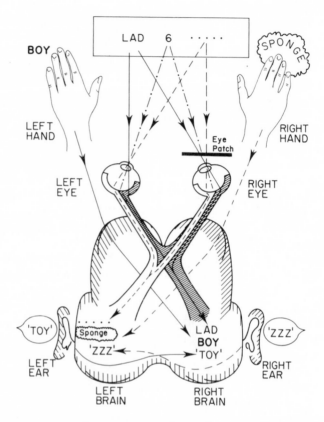

Correct response = '6 TOY'

Figure 6   Brain Function Therapy (BFT). Showing lateralized cross-tri-modal semantic discrimination task, where the
subject was required to discriminate between words presented simultaneously to the auditory, visual, and haptac
modalities. From Buffery, A. and Burton, A. (1982). Information processing and redevelopment: towards a science of
cognitive rehabilitation. In A. Burton (ed.), *Pathology and
Psychology of Cognition. Reproduced by permission of
Methuen and Co.*

left posterior temporal lesion. J.W. was discharged after over three years'
therapy and was considered to have maximized his recovery on the basis of his
clinician's judgement and assessment results. Extensive neuropsychological
assessment was carried out before the treatment programme began and
following each part of the programme. Tests included aphasia batteries, tests
of lateral preference for verbal material in each modality, and tests carried out
to eliminate visual, auditory and tactile agnosias, constructional apraxias, and
impaired tactile sensation. Results of initial assessment showed severe comprehension difficulty, mild semantic and phonemic paraphasia, and mild
anomia; a left lateral preference on two dichotic, two tachistoscopic, and two

haptic tests; no evidence of constructional or perceptual impairments in any modality, hemiparesis or visual-field defects.

A programme was designed to treat the subject's comprehension problem. This was based on current research evidence which suggests that phonemic discrimination (Luria, 1970; Blumstein, Baker, and Goodglass, 1977), an impairment in the processing of temporal aspects of speech (Albert and Bear, 1974; Tallal and Newcombe, 1978), and semantic discrimination (Boller, Kim, and Mack, 1977) are likely to underlie the comprehension loss in aphasia. It was reasoned that improved right hemisphere skills in phonemic discrimination, auditory verbal retention, and semantic discrimination for J.W. should produce improved comprehension and general communicative competence.

The treatment programme was in three parts: auditory–dichotic, visual–tachistoscopic and cross-modal. In Park I phonemic discrimination and auditory retention were treated using specially constructed dichotic tapes. The phonemic discrimination sub-programme involved the discrimination of dichotically presented pairs of CV syllables where the stop consonant differed in either voice, place or manner. J.W. was required to report verbally the syllable he heard in his left ear. Auditory verbal retention was treated using dichotically presented pairs of digits, increasing to three pairs of digits, heard with pauses reducing from 3 to 1.5 seconds between pairs. J.W. was asked to report as many left ear digits as he could. Finally in Part I, two increasing to three pairs of words were dichotically presented, with 3 decreasing to 2 seconds between pairs in a combined phonemic discrimination and auditory retention sub-programme. Here also, J.W. was expected to report the words he heard at his left ear.

In Part II letters, digits, and CVC words were tachistoscopically presented for identification and/or semantic discrimination. Geometric shapes were used at fixation in an attempt to 'prime' the right hemisphere (Kershner, Thomae, and Calloway, 1977). Letter presentation increased to three in each visual-field and digit presentation to four in each field as exposure time was systematically reduced. The subject had to identify as many letters or digits as possible in the left visual-field. CVC word discrimination built up to a three-word odd-one-out semantic discrimination task where J.W. was asked to state which of the three words (e.g., hat–bed–tie) was unrelated to the other two. Part III involved the cross-modal capabilities of dichotic and tachistoscopic presentation, where verbal auditory retention and phonemic discrimination were combined in a same/different paradigm. For instance, in one task J.W. was presented simultaneously with dichotic pairs of minimally paired words and words in the left visual-field for a same/different response.

The entire programme took about 19 months to work through and aphasia batteries and laterality tests were repeated following each of the three parts. Steady progress was observed during treatment and following each part of the programme with change on language tests showing modest but significant improvement in most areas. The laterality tests showed that there was a general increase in left ear and left visual-field preference during the programme causing an almost complete right ear and visual-field extinction by the end of the programme. Interestingly, although the haptic tests showed a left hand preference pre-treatment, this did not increase substantially during or following the programme but remained fairly stable throughout.

On the face of it, the results of both the BFT and HSR studies are encouraging. Both subjects—similar in many respects—made progress, apparently as a result of the programmes. Although Buffery's subject was apparently more severely aphasic than J.W., some eight or nine years older, and had suffered several CVAs, they were both patients who must be considered beyond any usual period of significant natural recovery. The results of aphasia and verbal IQ tests support the conclusion that improvement took place as a result of the programmes and detailed ongoing records of progress for J.W. would support such a conclusion. Whether the progress was due to a special form of direct right hemisphere stimulation or learning is another matter. For the moment, however, it might be noted that here is positive demonstration that improvement due to treatment can be demonstrated in aphasic patients, even in those who are beyond traditional conceptions of the spontaneous recovery period. Even this conclusion, however, is weakened by inadequate methodology in both studies.

As well as similarities, there are some interesting differences between the two studies which highlight some of the questions which remain. Buffery treated only via semantic discrimination and used a same/different paradigm throughout, whereas Code attempted to match treatment tasks as closely as possible to the patient's deficits in a patient-specific treatment programme. As concluded elsewhere in this book (Chapter 3), the right hemisphere appears to enjoy some semantic abilities and the treatment provided by Buffery could conceivably have built on a pre-existing semantic competence. However, the evidence also suggests that the normal right hemisphere has little competence in those tasks used by Code. Alternatively, therefore, as both patients appear to have made progress, then the precise nature of the linguistic stimuli directed to the right hemisphere may be unimportant. This might also support a general stimulation approach even to direct treatment of the right hemisphere: it may be the case that the right hemisphere can simply be prompted or encouraged to release latent linguistic abilities.

Unlike the BFT study, Code employed laterality tests to measure changes in lateral preference and reserved one modality as a control. Significant increase in left lateral preference was not observed in the control (tactile) modality during or following the programme, suggesting that increased left preference in the auditory and visual modalities was simply due to intense stimulation of left auditory and visual processes and was not a true reflection of *hemispheric* preference. This problem applies to both studies.

The rationale and aims of the two studies also differ somewhat. Buffery and Burton (1982) state:

BFT was designed (a) to monitor the damaged brain's ongoing patterns of functional recovery (BFT as 'probe'), and (b) to accelerate the rate of the damaged brain's functional recovery . . . (BFT as 'bombardment') (p. 274).

This would imply that a general stimulation approach was being adopted, although the authors describe BFT as 'influencing the course of relearning within the cerebrum' and focusing 'the learning process in one or other of the cerebral hemispheres' (p. 273). Thus although BFT and HSR aim to improve communication via increased right hemisphere involvement in language processing, the approach of HSR was designed actually to cause new learning rather than to act as bombardment. The gradual improvement in verbal abilities reported by both studies would tend to support a new learning rather than a wholesale linguistic shift hypothesis.

Despite the improvement shown by both patients, the methodological problems present in both studies make interpretation of results difficult. Firstly, was the observed improvement in the patients due to increased right hemisphere linguistic ability? As discussed in Chapter 2, the reliability of 'laterality tests' with brain damaged patients—especially ones with visual-field defects and hemiparesis—is so uncertain that their reliability in these studies must be suspect. Moreover, lateralizing techniques used in treatment can no longer be considered reliable and uncontaminated measures of hemispheric processing. Such measures taken with methods used in treatment may simply reflect an attentional bias induced by training. It is therefore clear that an uncontaminated control modality is necessary. Haptic measures taken during the HSR programme indicate that there was no increased involvement of the right hemisphere in verbal processing as a result of treatment, but future studies should consider reserving the visual modality as control as both haptic and dichotic responses can be more influenced by lesion effects. Neither study demonstrates that the improvements observed were due to an increased or enhanced verbal processing capability in the right hemisphere.

CONCLUSIONS

In this chapter we have been concerned to examine the role of the right hemisphere in the treatment of aphasia. Success has been reported in utilizing what appear to be the right hemisphere's compensatory strategies; but it is yet to be demonstrated that treatments designed to encourage more or swifter involvement of the right hemisphere in language processing actually have much influence.

While there is no harm in utilizing methods which may engage more right hemisphere involvement, and those involved in rehabilitation will always utilize theoretical knowledge and experimental findings in an intuitive and pragmatic manner, there is an absence of good evidence that the methods discussed achieve their aims—improved communication abilities beyond what might have been expected with other approaches. There is no shortage of creative ideas, but there is a shortage of evidence. This is partly due to the age-old problem of rehabilitation—measuring the effects of the *application* of theoretical predictions, laboratory findings, and large group averages to complex individual real-life situations. This is a complex problem which will not be solved easily. None the less, we should be constantly working towards improving the methods that we employ in measuring the effects of rehabilitation.

Some experimental methods have aimed more directly to access and manipulate right hemisphere processes and to re-establish lost abilities. The major question here is how much confidence can be placed in the assumption that the right hemisphere is actually (a) receiving the material directed to it via 'lateralizing' techniques; and (b) completing the tasks presented to it, and not passing them on to the left for processing? We have already seen that lesion effects hamper the application of lateralizing techniques with brain damaged subjects, and other methods are required to determine whether stimuli are reaching their targets. Bakker (Bakker, Moerland, and Goekoop-Hoefkens, 1981; Bakker and Vinke, 1985) has shown, in a pro-gramme aimed at improving reading skills in dyslexic children, that it is possible to use event-related potentials to determine whether tachistoscopi-cally presented words are reaching an intended hemisphere. This does not help with the problem stated in (b) above, however. There would appear to be no simple answer to this problem as techniques have not yet been developed which can reliably measure the neurophysiological concomitants of relatively complex linguistic stimuli in structured sessions.

However, much tighter designs could help answer this question. For instance, a crossover-treatment design (Coltheart, 1983b) could be used where the subject was tested on, for instance, dichotic and non-dichotic phonemic discrimination (Test 1), followed by dichotic treatment and retest in dichotic and non-dichotic conditions (Test 2). Treatment is then provided in the non-dichotic condition and both are tested again (Test 3). If the subject improves on dichotic testing in Test 2 but not in the non-dichotic condition, then this would indicate that improvement has taken place due to the specific effect of the dichotic presentation to the left ear. However, if improvement is seen in both conditions at Test 3, then this would indicate that improvement is not due to any special effect of unilateral presentation. In some hemispheric priming studies currently being conducted (Burton, Kemp, and Burton, 1985) attempts have been made to reduce some of the variance. An aphasic subject attends either to his left or right ear and reports when a match occurs between a dichotically presented object name and a line drawing. The indications so far for one subject are that such priming may impair rather than facilitate overall naming performance, but that left ear priming may improve naming of items failed at pre-test. The final results of these studies could help determine the clinical usefulness of direct hemispheric stimulation.

We have already concluded in previous chapters that the right hemisphere is involved in language processing in the normal brain and may take on extra responsibilities during the evolution of aphasia in some individuals. We have seen that attempts to use apparent right hemisphere processing to compensate for 'lost' language functions have been encouraging. Methods which aim to re-establish lost functions using more direct manipulation of cognitive processing need further careful research in order to demonstrate that they have any significant contribution to make to aphasia therapy.

Chapter Nine

CONCLUSIONS

In this final chapter we attempt to draw together some of the conclusions reached in previous chapters. The aim will be to present a summary sketch of current views on language processing in the right hemisphere. As illustrated throughout this volume, we are concerned with a rapidly developing field and firm conclusions are not possible in many areas.

In Chapter 2 we examined some of the major methodological problems in the area. Findings between studies are difficult to assess due to variation in quality of research, interpretation of data using different methodologies, and the wide range of populations studied. Failure of replication has hampered the development of neuropsychology. The evidence reviewed in Chapter 3 confirmed that the right hemisphere has substantial linguistic comprehension and Chapter 4 concluded that it may also enjoy a speech production capability, especially in more automatic, non-propositional aspects of speech production. Considering language beyond the narrow confines of the formal linguistic domain, the review presented in Chapter 5 suggested that the right hemisphere may play a major role in extralinguistic communication. Chapters 6 and 7 found evidence for right hemisphere involvement in language in aphasic individuals and Chapter 8 looked at the attempts to utilize this apparent involvement in rehabilitation.

In 1969 Bogen coined the term 'appositional' to describe the then relatively unknown form of processing of the right hemisphere. In less than two decades neuropsychological research has been able to place quite a lot of flesh on the bare bones of Bogen's appositional conception, and it is now widely considered that the right hemisphere cannot be considered the minor, subordinate or subservient hemisphere. Neurolinguistic research has spearheaded the reappraisal of the right hemisphere's role in cognition. The supremacy of the dominance model in modern neuropsychology was brought into question because clinical researchers began to observe that individuals with damage to the right side of the brain, could also have problems with language. At first many of these observations were explained away as secondary effects of impairment to what are seen as more primary modes, like visuospatial processing. Some right hemisphere symptoms, like the 'agraphia' observed following right hemisphere damage, can still be accounted for quite adequately in this way. But left hemisphere language is also highly dependent for its functioning on more fundamental cognitive processes. Although there is evidence to suggest that some kind of linguistic competence may be substantially preserved even in globally aphasic–apraxic patients (Glass, Gazzaniga, and Premack, 1973)—suggesting the autonomy of language—there is still a view that language could not have developed without the functional systems already existing, for bodily action for example (Kimura, 1973; Kimura and Archibald, 1974). It is not unreasonable to conclude therefore, that right hemisphere language also cannot exist in a vacuum, but owes its existence to basic information-processing forms.

We must start by stating that a comprehensive and integrated theory of the role of the right hemisphere in communication is not possible at this stage in our knowledge. None the less, as we have seen, researchers have proposed models to account for certain aspects of communication apparently mediated with right hemisphere involvement, although many are unhappy with attempts to subsume hemispheric differences in terms of opposing modes of processing. Whether the currently pursued complementary specialization model, and its main expression the analytic–holistic dichotomy, will continue to produce worthwhile research questions remains to be seen. Certainly, the notion that a cognitive balance is achieved by two fundamentally distinct methods of processing information is appealing. It is rooted in a long cultural, spiritual and scientific history, and may be the highest known expression of asymmetry that exists in nature.

We have seen some attempts at characterizing some aspects of right hemisphere language. There is, for instance, Jackson's proposal that non-propositional aspects of language are mediated with right hemisphere involvement, Wapner et al.'s (1981) model which holds that the right hemisphere has responsibility for certain complex, non-componential, context-dependent features of language, and Ross's suggestion that prosody is functionally and structurally represented in the right hemisphere, in the same way as formal linguistic aspects of language are traditionally considered to be represented in the left hemisphere. These and other models are currently at an early stage of development, and we have seen that many questions remain to be asked, and it is hoped, answered by future research.

Researchers have not been short of ideas. Characterizations of the contribution of the two hemispheres which have emerged from the research have been mainly in terms of complementary dichotomies, perhaps an almost inevitable and irresistible consequence of intense hemispheric differences research. In their discussion of the idea of hemisphericity, Beaumont, Young, and McManus (1984) have summarized the unease that many feel towards the dichotomous approach:

> It may in fact be the case that the idea that left- and right-hemisphere abilities can be described by any conceivable set of dichotomies will prove unworkable. Hemisphericity research is predicated on the view that suitable dichotomies can be found, because of three implicit assumptions. The first is that cerebral hemisphere differences are qualitative in nature. The second is that cerebral asymmetries reflect more general hemispheric asymmetries. The third is that these hemisphere differences exist because of fundamental incompatibilities

between different psychological processes, which need to be physically separated. All of these assumptions may be questioned (p. 204).

The unidimensional dominance idea, in contrast, is essentially a hierarchical model. Future research may work towards developing theories which attempt to combine features of both models into a more dynamic information-processing theory which takes into account the participation of non-cortical systems and processing capabilities in human communication, together with an improved consideration of the importance of individual differences. We no longer believe that 'language' is produced and comprehended by one or two discretely localized centres or mechanisms of the left hemisphere. These days we have a more humble appreciation of the complexities of human language and the mysteries of human brain. The future generation of investigatory techniques will produce more improved data on the involvement of subcortical systems in cognitive processes and their relationships with hemicortical mechanisms.

Any attempt to come up with a characterization of right hemisphere language at this time is bound to end up with the kind of list presented in Table 4. Here are brought together some of the findings, interpretations of findings, and proposed explanations into one table. Really, it represents a summary of the main topic of this book.

Following the improved intelligence gained in recent years on the impairments of communication which can follow right hemisphere damage, speech pathologists and clinical psychologists—mainly in the United States—are developing a clinical interest in the communication problems of the right-hemisphere-damaged. This has not yet resulted in a significant rehabilitation effort, although there is increased concern to devise assessment tools for clinical use. We are not yet in a position to construct a comprehensive or reliable 'right hemisphere language impairment battery', as our understanding of what to measure and how to measure it is still undergoing rapid change. However, Burns, Halper and Mogil (1985) have recently described a clinical evaluation of the communication of right hemisphere damaged patients. It provides tests and rating scales for anosognosia, orientation, visuoperceptual skills, intonation, writing, dialogue, narrative, and metaphor comprehension. Certain procedures based on the research already completed may prove useful in a clinical context.

For instance, the procedures used by Ross for his evaluation of prosodic impairment, semantic discrimination procedures like the ones devised by Gainotti and colleagues and Bishop and Bing and tests of complex linguistic entities and connotative meaning, might form the basis of some future battery. Many of the procedures used in the research summarized in Table 4 may prove useful in examining aspects of communication associated with right hemisphere damage. Those clinicians whose concern is with determining hemispheric side of damage through neuropsychological testing could usefully include in their evaluation some of the apparently more sensitive tests used in the research.

Table 4   Summary of Current Views on Right Hemisphere Language Capability

Apparent Underlying Processing Modes Visuospatial Gestalt–Holistic Ideographic	

Language Related Functions of Right Hemisphere *(some may be shared by left)*	*Chapter*
Emotional Processing	5
Musical Processing	5
Visuospatial Processing	1
Facial Expression	5

Models	*Chapter*
Non-propositional/Automatic Aspects of Speech (Jackson, 1874)	1,4
Non-literal, Pragmatic and Complex Linguistic Material (Wapner, Hamby, and Gardner, 1981)	5
Prosody (Ross, 1979)	5
Emotional Language (Bryden and Ley, 1983)	5
Facial Expression (Benton, 1980)	5

Possible Linguistic Functions of Right Hemisphere? *(some of which may be shared with left)*	*Chapter*
Auditory Comprehension	3
Semantic Discriminations	3
High Frequency, Imageable, Concrete Words	4
High Frequency, Concrete, Imageable and Visual Aspects of Reading	4,5
Visuospacial Aspects of Writing	4
More Acoustically Mediated Auditory Verbal Perception	7
Connotative, Non-referential Aspects of Meaning	3

We began this book from the position that the involvement of the right hemisphere in the processing of language and communication was not in question: the questions concerned the *extent* and the *nature* of that involvement. We have not been able to answer either question adequately. The dominant view is that the difference is quantitative and not qualitative (see commentaries to Bradshaw and Nettleton, 1981, for instance): the left hemisphere does more than the right, or what it does is more important. Logically, it does not have to be one or the other of course: left hemisphere processing involvement in some function may be qualitatively *and* quantitatively different to right hemisphere processing involvement in the same function. Part of the problem is the conflict in data from different samples as discussed in Chapter 2. The split-brain research, for instance, has been interpreted by some workers to support the view that the distinction is quantitative. It may be recalled that Sidtis *et al.* (1981) obtained results from commisurotomy patients V.P. and J.W. which showed a degree of language in V.P. and less in J.W. The right and left hemisphere capabilities of V.P. were interpreted to be qualitatively similar. However, the bilateral representation present from early life, as well as other criteria (i.e., early epilepsy, split-brain surgery), would indicate that what applies for V.P's. brain does not necessarily apply for other brains. Other split-brain workers (Zaidel, 1983; Zaidel and Schweiger, 1984) have interpreted the research to suggest a qualitative distinction between hemispheric capabilities in language.

Whether the hemispheres differ in the way they process information on a quantitive or a qualitative dimension, or both, remains an open question. The question may be ultimately unanswerable for the 'normal' population. Although average performances may be determinable on specific tasks, the indications we have suggest that right hemisphere language ability varies considerably, not only between different subgroups on tbe basis of sex, age, handedness, and occupation, but also between individuals. Furthermore, an individual's right hemisphere may vary its involvement in a specific task as a function of age, experience and training, task requirements, cognitive strategy choices, and even time of day. This has resulted in a return to the examination of the individual, especially the extraordinary individual.

The dominant information-processing paradigm of cognitive psychology has made a significant impact on neuropsychology in recent years. One major effect of this is to underscore the need to design research which will help to identify the information-processing stages involved when a human brain processes, transduces, transforms stimuli. Carmon (1981) has summed up the concern that is felt with regard to attempts to subsume the massive range of hemispheric differences findings into a neat bipolar characterization of any sort, rather than by a serious examination of the information-processing stages apparently employed by a given hemisphere in processing a stimulus:

> The only arbitrary or 'given' aspect of a stimulus is possibly that which is dependent on the way it is transduced. For example, a sound is always recognized by its temporal features. However, in higher stages the temporal features can be synthesized into acoustic patterns of timbre, chords, or pitch and further synthesized into higher-order melodic patterns. Spatial features can be synthesized into shapes of letters and words and then extracted by the left hemisphere in order to form a verbal sequence. Successive stages of processing thus allow for different modes of processing identical stimuli and a large degree of involvement of both hemispheres in cognitive processes (Carmon, 1981, p. 67).

A number of studies reviewed in earlier chapters have contributed detailed data on the processing stages involved in various activities. Oscar-Berman *et al.* (1978), for instance (see Chapter 2), have shown that asymmetries between hands can be produced by manipulating various processing stages in the perception and reporting of stimuli (digits, letters, and line orientations) 'drawn' on the palms of right-handed subjects. Tactile asymmetries only emerged on second report where the higher information-processing stages of memory—such as categorization, encoding, storage, and retrieval—appeared to be involved.

The problem is that some cognitive operations are more amenable to investigation of the stages of information processing than others. There is a danger, therefore, that some cognitive processes will be ignored by an approach which emphasizes those more easily characterizable operations. The synthesis of unitary or holistic information must be so much more complex, and hierarchically organized 'stages' are, by definition, not involved at all. As Marshall (1980, p. 72) has pointed out, the only explanation of how we recognize something as a Gestalt is that we recognize it as a Gestalt! Holistic synthesis, by definition, assumes a single stage of processing: something computers cannot, as yet, do. Holistic processing is not dependent upon previous, hierarchically earlier, stages of information processing. The fact that a form of processing is less accessible to present paradigms should not be confused to suggest that these forms of processing are less important. We must not fall into the trap of believing that the information-processing metaphor is some universal, God-given truth, any more than previous, pre-computer models were.

To some extent most branches of psychology are dependent upon technological and methodological developments for progress, and neuropsychology perhaps more than most. With future developments in methodology and technique our uncertainty of the role of the right hemisphere in communication and aphasia will reduce; maybe to the extent that we will be able to develop an improved understanding of its relationship with the rest of the central nervous system. The study of the effects of brain damage, especially resulting in aphasia, has contributed much to our understanding of brain–behaviour relationships and there are signs that work in aphasia recovery and rehabilitation is benefiting in like manner from neuropsychological research. An augmented knowledge of the right hemisphere's involvement in communication in the normal and damaged brain will contribute to the ultimate aim of neurolinguistics: an integrated understanding of the processing of language in the whole human brain.

REFERENCES

Abercrombie, D. (1968). Paralanguage. *British Journal of Disorders of Communication*, 3, 55-59.

Alajouanine, T. (1956). Verbal realization in aphasia. *Brain*, 79, 1-28.

Albert, M. L., and Bear, D. (1974). Time to understand: a case study in word deafness with reference to the role of time in auditory comprehension. *Brain*, 97, 373-384.

Albert, M. L., Sparks, R., and Helm, N. (1973). Melodic intonation therapy for aphasia. *Archives of Neurology*, 29, 130-131.

Alford, R. (1983). Sex differences in lateral facial facility: the effects of habitual emotional concealment. *Neuropsychologia*, 21, 567-569.

Alford, R., and Alford, K. F. (1981). Sex differences in asymmetry in the facial expression of emotion. *Neuropsychologia*, 19, 605-608.

Allen, J., and Haggard, M. (1977) Perception of voicing and place features in whispered speech: a dichotic choice analysis. *Perception and Psychophysics*, 21, 315-322.

Andy, O. J., and Bhatnagar, S. C. (1984). Right-hemispheric language evidence from cortical stimulation. *Brain and Language*, 23, 159-166.

Arseni, C., and Petrovici, I. N. (1971). Epilepsy in temporal lobe tumours. *European Neurology*, 5, 201-214.

Bailey, S. (1983). Blissymbolics and aphasia therapy: a case study. In: C. Code and D. Muller (eds.), *Aphasia Therapy*. London: Edward Arnold.

Bakan, P. (1969). Hypnotizability, laterality of eye movements and functional brain asymmetry. *Perceptual and Motor Skills*, 28, 927-932.

Bakan, P. (1980). Imagery, raw and cooked: a hemispheric recipe. In: J. E. Shorr, G. E. Sobel, P. Robin, and J. A. Connella (eds.), *Imagery: Its Many Dimensions and Applications*. New York: Plenum Press.

Bakan, P., and Shotland, L. (1969). Lateral eye movements, reading speed, and visual attention. *Psychonomic Science*, 15, 93-94.

Baker, E., Berry, T., Gardner, H., Zurif, E., Davis, L., and Veroff, A. (1975). Can linguistic competence be dissociated from natural language functions? *Nature*, 254, 509-510.

Bakker, D. J., Moerland, R., and Goekoop-Hoefkens, M. (1981). Effects of hemispheric stimulation on the reading performance of dyslexic boys: a pilot study. *Journal of Clinical Neuropsychology*, 3, 155-159.

Bakker, D. J., and Vinke, J. (1985). Effects of hemispheric-specific stimulation on brain activity and reading in dyslexics. *Journal of Clinical and Experimental Neuropsychology*, 7, 505-525.

Barton, M. I., Goodglass, H., and Shai, A. (1965). Differential recognition of tachistoscopically presented English and Hebrew words in right and left visual fields. *Perception and Motor Skills*, 21, 431-437.

Basser, L. S. (1962). Hemeplegia of early onset and the faculty of speech with special reference to the effects of hemispherectomy. *Brain*, 85, 427-460.

Beaumont, J. G. (1974). Handedness and hemispheric function. In: S. J. Dimond and J. G. Beaumont (eds.), *Hemispheric Function in the Human Brain*. London: Elek Science.

Beaumont, J. G. (ed.) (1982). *Divided Visual Field Studies of Cerebral Organization*. London: Academic Press.

Beaumont, J. G. (1983). *Introduction to Neuropsychology*. Oxford: Blackwells.

Beaumont, J. G., Young, A. W., and McManus, I. C. (1984). Hemisphericity: a critical review. *Cognitive Neuropsychology*, **1**, 191–212.

Benson, D., and Geschwind, N. (1975). The aphasias and related disturbances. In: A. B. Baker and L. D. Baker (eds.), *Clinical Neurology*. New York: Harper and Row.

Benson, D. F., Metter, E. J., Kuhl, D. E., and Phelps, M. E. (1983). Positron-computed tomography in neurobehavioral problems. In: A. Kertesz (ed.), *Localization in Neuropsychology*. London: Academic Press.

Benton, A. L. (1980). The neuropsychology of facial recognition. *American Psychologist*, **35**, 176–186.

Berg, M. R., and Harris, L. J. (1980). The effect of experimenter location and subject anxiety on cerebral activation as measured by lateral eye movements. *Neuropsychologia*, **18**, 89–93.

Berlin, C. I., and Cullen, J. K. Jr. (1977). Acoustic problems in dichotic listening tasks. In: S. J. Segalowitz and F. G. Gruber (eds.), *Language Developement and Neurological Theory*. New York: Academic Press.

Berlin, C. I., and McNeil, M. R. (1976). Dichotic Listening. In: N. J. Lass (ed.), *Contemporary Issues in Experimental Phonetics*. New York: Academic Press. 225–278.

Bever, T. G. (1983). Cerebral lateralization, cognitive asymmetry, and human consciousness. In: E. Perecman (ed.), *Cognitive Processing in the Right Hemisphere*. London. Academic Press.

Bever, T. G., and Chiarello, R. J. (1974). Cerebral dominance in musicians and nonmusicians. *Science*, **XX**, 137–139.

Beyn, E. S., and Shokhor-Trotskaya, M. K. (1966). The preventive method of speech rehabilitation in aphasia. *Cortex*, **2**, 96–108.

Bingley, H. (1958). Mental systems in temporal lobe epilepsy and temporal lobe gliomas. *Acta Psychiatrica et Neurologica Scandinavica*, **33**, Supplement 120.

Bishop, D., and Byng, S. (1984). Assessing semantic comprehension: methodological considerations and a new clinical test. *Cognitive Neuropsychology*, **1**, 233–244.

Blumstein, S., Baker, E., and Goodglass, H. (1977). Phonological factors in auditory comprehension in aphasia. *Neuropsychologica*, **15**, 19–30.

Blumstein, S., and Cooper, W. E. (1974). Hemispheric processing of intonation contours. *Cortex*, **10**, 146–157.

Blumstein, S., Goodglass, H., and Tartter, V. (1975). The reliability of ear advantage in dichotic listening. *Brain and Language*, **2**, 226–236.

Blunk, R., De Bleser, R., Willmes, K., and Zeumer, H. (1981). A refined method to relate morphological and functional aspects of aphasia. *European Neurology*, **30**, 68–79.

Bogen, J. E. (1969a). The other side of the brain. I: dysgraphia and dyscopia following cerebral commissurotomy. *Bulletin of the Los Angeles Neurological Societies*, **34**, 135–162.

Bogen, J. E. (1969b). The other side of the brain II: an appositional mind. *Bulletin of the Los Angeles Neurological Societies*, **34**, 135–162.

Bogen, J. E., and Bogen, G. M. (1969). The other side of the brain III: the corpus callosum and creativity. *Bulletin of the Los Angeles Neurological Societies*, **34**, 191–220.

Bogen, J. E., and Bogen, G. M. (1983). Hemispheric specialization and cerebral duality. *The Behavioral and Brain Sciences*, **3**, 517–520.

Bogen, J. E., DeZure, R., Houten, W. D., and Marsh, J. F. (1972). The other side of the brain IV: The A/P ratio. *Bulletin of the Los Angeles Neurological Societies*, **37**, 49–61.

Bogen, J. E., and Vogel, P. S. (1962). Cerebral commissurotomy in man. *Bulletin of the Los Angeles Neurological Societies*, **29**, 169–172.

Boller, F., Albert, M., and Denes, F. (1975). Pallilalia. *British Journal of Disorders of Communication*, **10**, 92–97.

Boller, F., Kim, Y., and Mack, J. L. (1977). Auditory comprehension in aphasia. In: H. and H. A. Whitaker (eds.), *Studies in Neurolinguistics*, Vol. 3. New York: Academic Press.

Borod, K. C., and Caron, H. S. (1980). Facedness and emotion related to lateral dominance, sex, and expression type. *Neuropsychologia*, **18**, 237–242.

Borod, J. C., and Goodglass, H. (1980). Lateralization of linguistic and melodic processing with age. *Neuropsychologia*, **18**, 79–83.

Borod, J. C., and Koff, E. (1983). Asymmetries in affective facial expression: behavior and anatomy. In: N. Fox and R. Davidson (eds.), *The Psychobiology of Affective Development*. Philadelphia: Erlbaum and Associates.

Borod, J. C., Koff, E., and Caron, H. S. (1983a). Right hemisphere specialization for the expression and appreciation of emotion: a focus on the face. In: E. Perecman (ed.), *Cognitive Processing in the Right Hemisphere*. London: Academic Press.

Borod, J. C., Koff, E., and White, B. (1983b). Facial asymmetry in posed and spontaneous expressions of emotion. *Brain and Cognition*, **2**, 165–175.

Bradshaw, J. L. (1980). Right hemisphere language: familial and nonfamilial sinistrals, cognitive deficits and writing hand position in sinistrals, and the concrete–absract, imageable–nonimageable dimensions in word recognition. A review of interrelated issues. *Brain and Language*, **10**, 172–185.

Bradshaw, J. L., and Gates, A. (1978). Visual field differences in verbal tasks: effects of task familiarity and sex of subject. *Brain and Language*, **5**, 166–187.

Bradshaw, J. L., and Nettleton, N. C. (1981). The nature of hemispheric specialization in man. *The Behavioural and Brain Sciences*, **4**, 51–91.

Bradshaw, J. L., and Taylor, M. J. (1979). A word-naming deficit in nonfamilial sinistrals? Laterality effects of vocal responses to tachistoscopically presented letter strings. *Neuropsychologia*, **17**, 21–32.

Brady, W. A. (1978). Auditory and visual response patterns of right and left temporo-parietal lobe damaged patients for linguistic and non-linguistic stimuli. Unpublished Ph.D. Thesis, Kent State University.

Briggs, G. G., and Nebes, R. D. (1976). The effects of handedness, family history and sex on performance of a dichotic listening task. *Neuropsychologia*, **14**, 129–134.

Broadbent, D. E. (1954). The role of auditory localization in attention and memory. *Journal of Experimental Psychology*, **47**, 191–196.

Broca, P. (1861). Remarques sur le siege de la faculté du langage articulé suivies d'une observation d'aphemie (perte de la parole). *Paris Bulletin de la Société d'Anatomie*, **36**, 330–357.

Broca, P. (1865). Du siege de la faculté de langage articulé. *Bulletin de la Société d'Anthropologie*, **6**, 337–393.

Brown, J. W. (1975). On the neural representation of language: thalmic and cortical relationships. *Brain and Language*, **2**, 18–30.

Brown, J. W. (1976). Consciousness and the pathology of language. In: R. W. Rieber (ed.), *The Neuropsychology of Language*. New York: Plenum Press.

Brown, J. W. (1979). Language representation in the brain. In: H. D. Steklis and M. J. Raleigh (eds.), *Neurobiology of Social Communication in Primates*. New York: Academic Press.

Brown, J. W. (1981). Introduction. In J. W. Brown (ed.), *Jargonaphasia*. New York: Academic Press.

Brown, J. W., and Jaffe, J. (1975). Hypothesis on cerebral dominance. *Neuropsychologia*, **13**, 107–110.

Brunner, R. J., Kornhuber, H. H., Seemuller, E., Sugar, G., and Wallesch, C-W. (1982). Basal ganglia participation in language pathology. *Brain and Language*, **16**, 281–299.

Bryden, M. P. (1963). Ear preference in auditory perception. *Journal of Experimental Psychology*, **65**, 103–105.

Bryden, M. P. (1965). Tachistoscopic recognition, handedness, and cerebral dominance. *Neuropsychologia*, **3**, 1–8.

Bryden, M. P. (1966). Left–right differences in tachistoscopic recognition: directional scanning or cerebral dominance? *Perceptual and Motor Skills*, **23**, 1127–1134.

Bryden, M. P. (1973). Perceptual asymmetry in vision: relation to handedness, eyedness, and speech lateralization. *Cortex*, **9**, 418–435.

Bryden, M. P. (1978). Strategy effects in the assessment of hemispheric assymmetry. In G. Underwood (ed.), *Strategies of Information Processing*. London: Academic Press.

Bryden, M. P., and Allard, F. (1978). Dichotic listening and the development of linguistic processes. In M. Kinsbourne (ed.), *Asymmetrical Function of the Brain*. Cambridge: Cambridge University Press.

Bryden, M. P., and Ley, R. G. (1983). Right hemisphere involvement in imagery and effect. In: E. Perecman (ed.), *Cognitive Processing in the right Hemisphere*. London: Academic Press.

Bryden, M. P., Ley, G., and Sugarman, J. H. (1982). A left-ear advantage for identifying the emotional quality of tonal sequences. *Neuropsychologia*, **20**, 83–87.

Bryer, R. (1981). Asymmetry of facial expression in brain damaged subjects. *Neuropsychologia*, **19**, 615–624.

Buck, R., and Duffy, R. J. (1980). Nonverbal communication of affect in brain-damaged patients. *Cortex*, **16**, 351–362.

Buffery, A. W. (1977). Clinical neuropsychology; review and preview. In S. Rachman (ed.), *Contributions to Medical Psychology*: Vol. I. Oxford: Pergamon Press.

Buffery, A. W., and Burton, A. (1982). Information processing and redevelopment: towards a science of cognitive rehabilitation. In: A. Burton (ed.), *Pathology and Psychology of Cognition*. London: Methuin.

Burton, A., Kemp, R. I., and Burton, K. (1986). Hemispheric priming and picture naming in aphasics. Research Report, Department of Psychology, North East London Polytechnic.

Butler, S. R., and Norrsell, U. (1968). Vocalization possibly initiated by the minor hemisphere. *Nature*, **220**, 793–794.

Campbell, R. (1978). Asymmetries in interpreting and expressing a posed facial expression. *Cortex*, **14**, 327–342.

Cannezzio, L. (1977). The effects of visual coding, word frequency and word imageability on aphasic's word-matching abilities. Master's Thesis; Hunter College, City University, New York.

Caplan, L., and Hedley-White, T. (1974). Cueing and memory disfunction in alexia without agraphia. *Brain*, **97**, 251–262.

Caramazza, A. (1984). The logic of neuropsychological research and the problem of patient classification in aphasia. *Brain and Language*, **21**, 9–29.

Carmon, A. (1981). Temporal processing and the left hemisphere. *The Behavioral and Brain Sciences*, **4**, 66–67.

Carmon, A., and Nachshon, I. (1973). Ear asymmetry in perception of emotional non-verbal stimuli. *Acta Psychologia*, **37**, 351–357.

Carrier, J. (1974). Non speech noun usage training with severely and profoundly retarded children. *Journal of Speech and Hearing Disorders*, **17**, 510–517.

Carrier, J., and Peak, T. (1974). Non Speech Language Initiation Program. Lawrence, Kansas: H. & H. Enterprises.

Castro-Caldas, A., and Botelho, M. A. S. (1980). Dichotic listening in the recovery of aphasia after stroke. *Brain and Language*, **10**, 145–151.

Cavalli, M., DeRenzi, E., Faglioni, P., and Vitali, A. (1981). Impairment of right brain-damaged patients on a linguistic cognitive task. *Cortex*, **17**, 545–556.

Chase, R. A., Cullen, J. K., Niedermeyer, E. F., Stark, R. E., and Blumer, D. P. (1967). Ictal speech automatisms and swearing: studies on the auditory feedback control of speech. *The Journal of Nervous and Mental Disease*, **144**, 406–420.

Cicone, M., Warner, W., and Gardner, H. (1980). Sensitivity to emotional expressions and situations by organic patients. *Cortex*, **16**, 145–158.

Code, C. (1981). Dichotic listening with the communicatively impaired: results from trials of a short British-English dichotic word test. *Journal of Phonetics*, **9**, 375–383.

Code, C. (1982a). Neurolinguistic analysis of recurrent utterances in aphasia. *Cortex*, **18**, 141–152.

Code, C. (1982b). On the origins of recurrent utterances in aphasia. *Cortex*, **18**, 161–164.

Code, C. (1983a). On 'Neurolinguistic analysis of recurrent utterances in aphasia': reply to de Bleser and Poeck. *Cortex*, **19**, 259–264.

Code, C. (1983b). The validity of dichotic listening as an indicator of hemispheric shift in aphasia: dominance vs. lesion effects in the performance of fluent and nonfluent subjects. Paper presented at Dysphasia Conference, Middlesex Hospital, London.

Code, C. (1983c). Hemispheric specialization retraining: possibilities and problems. In: Code and D. J. Muller (eds.), *Aphasia Therapy*. London: Edward Arnold.

Code, C. (1984a). Dichotic listening. In: C. Code and M. J. Ball (eds.), *Experimental Clinical Phonetics*. Beckenham: Croom Helm.

Code, C. (1984b). Delayed auditory feedback. In: C. Code and M. J. Ball (eds.), *Experimental Clinical Phonetics*. Beckenham: Croom Helm.

Code, C. (1986). Catastrophic reaction and anosognosia in anterior–posterior and left–right models of the cerebral control of emotion. *Psychological Research*, **48**, 53–55.

Code, C., and Ball, M. J. (eds.) (1984). *Experimental Clinical Phonetics*. Beckenham: Croom Helm.

Cohen, G. (1977). *The Psychology of Cognition*. London: Academic Press.

Coltheart, M. (1980a). Deep dyslexia: a right hemisphere hypothesis. In: M. Coltheart, K. Patterson, and J. C. Marshall (eds.), *Deep Dyslexia*. London: Routledge and Kegan Paul.

Coltheart, M. (1980b). Deep dyslexia: a review of the syndrome. In: M. Coltheart, K. Patterson, and J. C. Marshall (eds.), *Deep Dyslexia*. London: Routledge and Kegan Paul.

Coltheart, M. (1983a). The right hemisphere and disorders of reading. In: A. Young (ed.), *Functions of the Right Cerebral Hemisphere*. London: Academic Press.

Coltheart, M. (1983b). Researching into aphasia therapy: the single-case study approach. In: C. Code and D. J. Muller (eds.), *Aphasia Therapy*. London Edward Arnold.

Coltheart, M., Patterson, K., and Marshall, J. C. (eds.) (1983). *Deep Dyslexia*. London: Routledge and Kegan Paul.

Cooper, R., Ossleton, J. W., and Shaw, J. C. (1980). *EEG Technology* (3rd Edition). London: Butterworth.

Critchley, M. (1953). *The Parietal Lobes*. London: Edward Arnold.

Critchley, M. (1970). *Aphasiology and Other Aspects of Language*. London: Edward Arnold.

Crockett, H. G., and Estridge, N. M. (1951). Cerebral hemispherectomy. *Bulletin of the Los Angeles Neurological Societies*, **16**, 71–87.

Crosson, B., and Warren, R. L. (1981). Dichotic ear preferences for C-V-C words in Wernicke's and Broca's aphasia. *Cortex*, **17**, 249–258.

Crystal, D. (1969). *Prosodic Systems and Intonation in English*. Cambridge: Cambridge University Press.

Culton, G. (1969). Spontaneous recovery from aphasia. *Journal of Speech and Hearing Research*, **12**, 825–832.

Cummings, J. L., Benson, J. L., Walsh, M. J., and Levine, H. L. (1979). Left-to-right transfer of language dominance: a case study. *Neurology*, **29**, 1547–1550.

Curry, F. K. W. (1967). A comparison of left-handed and right-handed subjects on verbal and non-verbal dichotic listening tasks. *Cortex*, **3**, 343–352.

Cutler, A., and Isard, S. D. (1980). The production of prosody. In: B. Butterworth (ed.), *Language Production*: Volume 1; *Speech and Talk*. London: Academic Press.

Czopf, C. (1972). Uber die Rolle der nicht dominanten Hemisphere in der restitution der Sprache der Aphasischen. *Arch. Psychiat. Nervenkr.*, **216**, 162–171.

Czopf, C. (1979). The role of the non-dominant hemisphere in speech recovery in aphasia. *Aphasia-Apraxia-Agnosia*, **1**, 27–33.

Damasio, H., and Damasio, A. R. (1979). 'Paradoxic' extinction in dichotic listening: possible anatomic significance. *Neurology*, **29**, 644–653.

Danly, M., Cooper, W. E., and Shapiro, B. (1983). Fundamental frequency, language processing, and linguistic structure in Wernicke's aphasia. *Brain and Language*, **19**, 1–24.

Danly, M., and Shapiro, B. (1982). Speech prosody in Broca's aphasia. *Brain and Language*, **16**, 171–190.

Darley, F. L., Aronson, A. E., and Brown, J. R. (1975). *Motor Speech Disorders*. Philadelphia: Saunders.

Darwin, C. J. (1971). Ear differences in the recall of fricatives and vowels. *Quarterly Journal of Experimental Psychology*, **23**, 46–62.

Darwin, C. J. (1974). Ear differences and hemispheric specialization. In: F. O. Schmidt and F. Worden (eds.), *The Neurosciences*, Vol. III. Cambridge Massachusetts: MIT Press.

Davidson, R., and Schwartz, G. (1976). Patterns of cerebral lateralization during cardiac biofeedback versus the self-regulation of emotion. *Psychophysiology*, **13**, 62–74.

Davis, G. A., and Holland, A. L. (1981). Age in understanding and treating aphasia. In: D. S. Beasley and G. A. Davis (eds.), *Aging: Communication Processes and Disorders*. New York: Grune and Stratton.

Davis, G. A., and Wilcox, M. J. (1981). Incorporating parameters of natural conversation in aphasia treatment. In: R. Chapey (ed.), *Language Intervention Strategies in Adult Aphasia*. Baltimore: Williams and Wilkins.

Davis, G. A., and Wilcox, M. J. (1985). *Adult Aphasia Rehabilitation: Applied Pragmatics*. Windsor: NFER–Nelson.

Dax, M. (1865). Lesions de la moitie gauche de l'encephale coincident avec l'oubli des signes de la pensee. *Montpeliere Gazzette Hebdom adaire*, (1836), **11**, 259–260.

Day, J. (1977). Right-hemisphere language processing in normal right-handers. *Journal of Experimental Psychology: Human Perception and Performance*, **3**, 518–528.

De Bleser, R., and Poeck, K. (1983). Comments on paper 'Neurolinguistic analysis of recurrent utterances in aphasia' by C. Code. *Cortex*, **19**, 259–260.

De Bleser, R., and Poeck, K. (1985). Analysis of prosody in the spontaneous speech of patients with CV-recurring utterances. *Cortex*, **21**, 405–416.

DeKosky, S. T., Heilman, K. M., Bowers, D., and Valenstein, E. (1980). Recognition and discrimination of emotional faces and pictures. *Brain and Language*, **9**, 206–214.

Dennis, M., and Whitaker, H. A. (1976). Language acquisition following hemidecortication: linguistic superiority of left over right hemisphere. *Brain and Language*, **3**, 404–433.

DeRenzi, E. (1977). Hemispheric asymmetry as evidence of spatial disorders. In: M.

Kinsbourne (ed.), *Asymmetrical Function of the Brain*. Cambridge: Cambridge University Press.

DeRenzi, E., Faglioni, P., and Ferrari, P. (1980). The influence of sex and age on the incidence and type of aphasia. *Cortex*, **16**, 627–630.

Dimond, S. J., Bures, J., Farrington, I. J., and Broawers, E. Y. M. (1975). The use of contact lenses for the localization of visual input in man. *Acta Psychologica*, **39**, 341–349.

Dimond, S. J. and Farrington, L. (1977). Emotional response to films shown to right or left hemisphere of the brain measured by heart rate. *Acta Psychologica*, **41**, 255–260.

Dimond, S. J., Farrington, L., and Johnson, P. (1976). Differing emotional response from right and left hemisphere. *Nature*, **261**, 689–691.

DiSimoni, F. G. (1981). Therapies which utilize alternative or augmentative communication systems. In: R. Chapey (ed.), *Language Intervention Strategies in Adult Aphasia*. Baltimore: Williams and Wilkins.

Dobson, W. G., Beckwith, B. E., Tucker, D. M., and Bullard-Bates, D. C. (1984). Asymmetry of facial expression in spontaneous emotion. *Cortex*, **20**, 243–251.

Dordain, M., Degos, J. D., and Dordain, G. (1971). Troubles de la voix dans les hemiplegies gauches. *Review of Laryngology, Otolaryngology and Rhinology*, **92**, 178–188.

Duda, P. D. and Brown, J. (1984). Lateral asymmetry of positive and negative emotions. *Cortex*, **20**, 253–261.

Duke, J. (1968). Lateral eye movement behaviour. *Journal of General Psychology*, **78**, 189–195.

Eccles, J. C. (1965). *The Brain and the Unity of Conscious Experience*. London: Cambridge University Press.

Eccles, J. C. (1973). *The Understanding of the Brain*. New York: McGraw-Hill.

Eccles, J. C. (1977). Evolution of the brain in relation to the development of the self-conscious mind. In: S. J. Dimond and D. A. Blizard (eds.), *Evolution and Lateralization of the Brain*. Annals of the New York Academy of Sciences, **229**, 161–179.

Edelstein, D. (1977). Visual imagery and recognition memory in aphasia. Master's Thesis, Hunter College, City University, New York.

Efron, R., and Yund, E. W. (1974). Dichotic competition of simultaneous tone bursts of different frequency 1. Dissociation of pitch from lateralization and loudness. *Neuropsychologia*, **12**, 249–256.

Eisenson, J. (1962). Language and intellectual modification associated with right cerebral damage. *Language and Speech*, **5**, 49–53.

Eisenson, J. (1964). Discussion. In: A. V. S. DeReuck and M. O'Conner (eds.), *Disorders of Language*. London: Churchill.

Eisenson, J. (1981). Issues, prognosis, and problems in the rehabilitation of language disorders in adults. In: R. Chapey (ed.), *Language Intervention Strategies in Adult Aphasia*. Baltimore: Williams and Wilkins.

Ekman, P., Hager, J., and Friesen, W. (1981). The asymmetry of emotional and deliberate facial action. *Psychophysiology*, **18**, 101–106.

Ellis, H. D., and Sheppard, J. W. (1974). Recognition of abstract and concrete words presented in right and left visual field. *Journal of Experimental Psychology*, **103**, 1035–1036.

Ellis, H. D., and Shepherd, J. W. (1975). Recognition of upright and inverted faces presented to the left and right visual fields. *Cortex*, **11**, 3–7.

Enderby, P., and Hamilton, G. (1983). Communication aid and therapeutic tool: a report on the clinical trial using Splink with aphasic patients. In: C. Code and D. Muller (eds.), *Aphasia Therapy*. London: Edward Arnold.

Falconer, M. A. (1967). Brain mechanisms suggested by neurophysiologic studies. In:

C. H. Millikan and F. L. Darley (eds.), *Brain Mechanisms Underlying Speech and Language*. New York: Grune and Stratton.

Foldi, N. S., Cicone, M., and Gardner, H. (1983). Pragmatic aspects of communication in brain-damaged patients. In: S. J. Segalowitz (ed.). *Language Functions and Brain Organization*. New York: Academic Press.

Fried, I., Matser, C., Ojemann, G., Wohms, R., and Fedio, P. (1982). Organization of visuospatial functions in human cortex. *Brain*, 105, 349–371.

Frumkin, L. R., Ripley, H. S., and Cox, G. B. (1978). Changes in cerebral hemispheric lateralization with hypnosis. *Biological Psychiatry*, 13, 741–750.

Gainotti, G. (1969). Reactions 'catastrophic' et manifestations d'indifference au cours des atteintes cerebrales. *Neuropsychologia*, 7, 195–204.

Gainotti, G. (1972). Emotional behaviour and hemispheric side of the lesion. *Cortex*, 8, 41–55.

Gainotti, G., Caltagirone, C., and Miceli, G. (1979). Semantic disorders of auditory language comprehension in right brain-damaged patients. *Journal of Psycholinguistic Research*, 8, 13–20.

Gainotti, G., Caltagirone, C., and Miceli, G. (1983). Selective impairment of semantic-lexical discrimination in right-brain-damaged patients. In: E. Perecman (ed.), *Cognitive Processing in the Right Hemisphere*. London: Academic Press.

Gainotti, G., Caltagirone, C., Miceli, G., and Masullo, C. (1981). Selective semantic–lexical impairment of language comprehension in right-brain-damaged patients. *Brain and Language*, 13, 201–211.

Galin, D., Diamond, R., and Braff, D. (1977). Lateralization of conversion symptoms: more frequent on the left. *American Journal of Psychiatry*, 134, 578–580.

Gardner, H. (1982). Artistry following damage to the human brain. In: A. Ellis (ed.), *Normality and Pathology in Cognitive Functions*. London: Academic Press.

Gardner, H., Brownell, H. H., Wapner, W., and Michelow, D. (1983). Missing the point: the role of the right hemisphere in the processing of complex linguistic materials. In: E. Perecman (ed.), *Cognitive Processing in the Right Hemisphere*. London: Academic Press.

Gardner, H., Zurif, E. B., Berry, T., and Baker, E. (1976). Visual communication in aphasia. *Neuropsychologia*, 11, 95–103.

Gazzaniga, M. S. (1970). *The Bisected Brain*. New York: Appleton-Century Crofts.

Gazzaniga, M. S. (1974a). Cerebral dominance viewed as a decision making system. In: S. J. Dimond and J. G. Beaumont (eds.), *Hemispheric Function in the Human Brain*. London: Elek Science.

Gazzaniga, M. S. (1974b). Determinants of cerebral recovery. In: D. G. Stein, J. J. Rosen, and N. Butters (eds.), *Plasticity and Recovery of Function in the Central Nervous System*. London: Academic Press.

Gazzaniga, M. S. (1977). Consistency and diversity in brain organization. *Annals of the New York Academy of Sciences*, 299, 415–423.

Gazzaniga, M. S. (1983). Right hemisphere language following brain bisection: a 20-year perspective. *American Psychologist*, 38, 525–537.

Gazzaniga, M. S., Bogen, J. E., and Sperry, R. W. (1962). Some functional effects of sectioning the cerebral commissures in man. *Proceedings of the National Academy of Sciences*, 48, 1765–1769.

Gazzaniga, M. S., Bogen, J. E., and Sperry, R. W. (1963). Laterality effects in somesthesis following cerebral commissurotomy in man. *Neuropsychologia*, 1, 209–215.

Gazzaniga, M. S., and Hillyard, S. A. (1971). Language and speech capacity of the right hemisphere. *Neuropsychologia*, 9, 273–380.

Gazzaniga, M. S., and LeDoux, J. E. (1978). *The Integrated Mind*. New York: Plenum Press.

180

Gazzaniga, M. S., LeDoux, J. E., and Wilson, D. H. (1977). Language, praxis, and the right hemisphere: clues to some mechanisms of consciousness. *Neurology*, 27, 1144–1147.

Gazzaniga, M. S., Risse, G. L., Springer, S P., Clark, R., and Wilson, D. H. (1975). Psychological and neurologic consequences of partial and complete commissurotomy. *Neurology (Minneap)*, 25, 10–15.

Gazzaniga, M. S., Smylie, C. S., Baynes, K., Hirst, W., and McCleary, C. (1984). Profiles of right hemisphere language and speech following brain bisection. *Brain and Language*, 22, 206–220.

Gazzaniga, M. S., and Sperry, R. W. (1967). Language after sectioning of the cerebral commissures. *Brain*, 90, 131–148.

Gazzaniga, M. S., Volpe, B. T., Smylie, C. S., Wilson, D. H. and LeDoux, J. E. (1979). Plasticity in speech organization following commissurotomy. *Brain*, 102, 805–815.

Geschwind, N. (1965a). Disconnection syndromes in animals and man: Part I. *Brain*, 88, 237–294.

Geschwind, N. (1965b). Disconnection syndromes in animals and man: Part II. *Brain*, 88, 585–646.

Geschwind, N. (1974). Late changes in the nervous system; an overview. In: D. G. Stein, J. J. Rosen, and N. Butters (eds.) *Plasticity and Recovery of Function in the Central Nervous System*. London: Academic Press.

Glass, A. V., Gazzaniga, M. S., and Premack, D. (1973). Artificial language training in global aphasics. *Neuropsychologia*, 11, 95–103.

Gloning, I., Gloning, K., Haube, G., and Quatember, R. (1969). Comparison of verbal behavior in right-handed and non-right-handed patients with anatomically verified lesion of one hemisphere. *Cortex*, 5, 41–52.

Gloning, K., Trappl, R., Heiss, W. D., and Quatember, R. (1976). Prognosis and speech therapy in aphasia. In: Y. Lebrun and R. Hoops (eds.) *Recovery in Aphasia*. Amsterdam(Swets and Zeitlinger.

Goldstein, G. (1974). The use of clinical neuropsychological methods in the lateralization of brain lesions. In: S. J. Dimond and J. G. Beaumont (eds.), *Hemispheric Function in the Human Brain*. London: Elec Science.

Goldstein, K. (1948). *Language and Language Disturbances*. New York: Grune and Stratton.

Goldman-Eisler, F. (1968). *Psycholinguistics: Experiments in Spontaneous Speech*. London: Academic Press.

Gombrich, E. N. (1968). *Art and Illusion: a Study in the Psychology of Pictorial Representation*. London: Phaidon Press.

Goodglass, H., and Geschwind, N. (1976). Language disorders (aphasia). In: E. C. Carterette and M. P. Friedman (eds.), *Handbook of Perception*, Vol. VII: *Language and Speech*. New York: Academic Press.

Goodglass, H., and Peck, E. A. (1972). Dichotic ear order effects in Korsakoff and normal subjects. *Neuropsychologia*, 10, 211–217.

Gordon, H. W. (1970) Hemispheric asymmetries in the perception of musical chords. *Cortex*, 6, 387–396.

Gordon, H. W. (1975). Hemispheric asymmetries and musical performance. *Science*, 189, 68–69.

Gordon, H. W. (1978). Hemispheric asymmetry for dichotically presented chords in musicians and non-musicians, males and females. *Acta Psychologia*, 42, 383–395.

Gordon, H. W. (1980). Right hemisphere comprehension of verbs in patients with complete forebrain commissurotomy: use of the dichotic method and manual performance. *Brain and Language*, 11, 76–86.

Gowers, W. R. (1887). *Lectures in the Diagnosis of Diseases of the Brain*. Philadelphia: P. Blakiston.

Graves, R. (1983). Mouth asymmetry, dichotic ear advantage and tachistoscopic visual field advantage as measures of language lateralization. *Neuropsychologia*, **21**, 641–649.

Graves, R., Landis, T., and Goodglass, H. (1981). Laterality and sex differences for visual recognition of emotional and non-emotional words. *Neuropsychologia*, **19**, 95–102.

Graves, R., Landis, T., and Goodglass, H. (1982). Mouth asymmetry during spontaneous speech. *Neuropsychologia*, **20**, 371–381.

Gregory, A. H. (1982). Ear dominance for pitch. *Neuropsychologia*, **20**, 89–90.

Gross, M. M. (1972). Hemispheric specialization for processing of visually presented verbal and spatial stimuli. *Perception and Psychophysics*, **12**, 357–363.

Gur, R., and Gur, R. E. (1974). Handedness, sex, and eyedness as moderating variables in the relation between hypnotic susceptibility and functional brain asymmetry. *Journal of Abnormal Psychology*, **83**, 635.

Gur, R. E., Gur, R. C., and Harris, L. J. (1975). Cerebral activation, as measured by subject's lateral eye movements, is influenced by experimenter location. *Neuropsychologia*, **13**, 33–44.

Haggard, M. P. (1971). Encoding and the REA for speech signals. *Quarterly Journal of Experimental Psychology*, **23**, 34–45.

Haggard, M. P., and Parkinson, A. M. (1971). Stimulus and task factors as determinants of ear advantages. *Quarterly Journal of Experimental Psychology*, **23**, 168–177.

Hannay, H. J. and Malone, P. R. (1976). Visual field effects and short-term memory for verbal material. *Neuropsychologia*, **14**, 203–209.

Hardyck, C., and Petrinovitch, L. F. (1977). Left-handedness. *Psychological Bulletin*, **44**, 385–404.

Harris, L. J. (1980). Which hand is the 'eye' of the blind? A new look at an old question. In: J. Herron (ed.), *Neuropsychology of Left Handedness*. New York: Academic Press.

Harris, L. J., and Carr, T. H. (1983). Implications of differences between perceptual systems for analysis of hemispheric specialization. *The Behavioral and Brain Sciences*, **4**, 71–72.

Hatta, T. (1977). Recognition of Japanese kanji in the left and right visual field. *Neuropsychologia*, **15**, 685–688.

Hatta, T. (1978). Recognition of Japanese kanji in hirakana in the left and right visual fields. *Japanese Psychological Research*, **20**, 51–59.

Hayden, M. E., Kirsten, E., and Singh, S. (1979). Role of distinctive features in dichotic presentation of 21 English consonants. *Journal of the Acoustical Society of America*, **65**, 1039–1046.

Head, H. (1926). *Aphasia and Kindred Disorders of Speech*. Cambridge: Cambridge University Press.

Hécaen, H., and Albert, M. L. (1978). *Human Neuropsychology*. New York: John Wiley and Sons.

Hécaen, H., and Angelergues, R. (1960). Epilepsie et troubles du langage. *Encephale*, **49**, 138–169.

Hécaen, H., and Marcie, P. (1974). Disorders of written language following right hemisphere lesions: spatial dysgraphia. In: S. J. Dimond and J. G. Beaumont (ed.), *Hemispheric Function in the Human Brain*. London: Elek.

Hécaen, H., and Sauguet, J. (1971). Cerebral dominance in left-handed subjects. *Cortex*, **7**, 19–48.

Heilman, K. M., Scholes, R., and Watson, R. T. (1976). Auditory affective agnosia. *Journal of Neurology, Neurosurgery and Psychiatry*, **38**, 69–72.

Heilman, K. M., Watson, R. T., Valenstein, E., and Damasio, A. R. (1983). Localization of lesion in neglect. In: A. Kertesz (ed.), *Localization in Neuropsychology*. London: Academic Press.

Helm-Easterbrook, N., FitzPatrick, P. M., and Barresi, B. (1982). Visual Action Therapy for global aphasia. *Journal of Speech and Hearing Disorders*, **47**, 385–389.

Henschen, S. E. (1922). *Klinische und anatomische Beitrage zur Pathologie des Gehirns* (Vols. 5–7). Stockholm: Wordiska Bokhondel'n.

Hicks, R. (1975). Intrahemispheric response competition between vocal and unimanual performance in normal adult human males. *J. Comp. Physiol. Psychol.*, **89**, 50–60.

Hicks, R. F., and Kinsbourne, M. (1978). Handedness differences: human handedness. In: M. Kinsbourne (ed.), *The Asymmetrical Function of the Brain*. New York: Cambridge University Press.

Hier, D. B., and Kaplan, J. (1980). Verbal comprehension deficits after right hemisphere damage. *Applied Psycholinguistics*, **1**, 279–294.

Hillier, W. F. (1954). Total left cerebral hemispherectomy for malignant glioma. *Neurology*, **4**, 718–721.

Hines, D. (1972). A brief reply to McKeever, Suberi and Van Deventer's comments on 'Bilateral tachistoscopic recognition of verbal and nonverbal stimuli'. *Cortex*, **8**, 480–482.

Hines, D. (1976). Recognition of verbs, abstract nouns and concrete nouns from the left and right visual half fields. *Neuropsychologia*, **14**, 211–216.

Hines, D. (1977). Differences in tachistoscopic recognition between abstract and concrete words as a function of visual half-field and frequency. *Cortex*, **13**, 66–73.

Hirshkowitz, M., Earle, J., and Paley, B. (1978). EEG alpha asymmetry in musicians and nonmusicians. A study of hemispheric specialization. *Neuropsychologia*, **16**, 125–128.

Holland, A. (1980). *Communicative Activities in Daily Living*. Baltimore: University Park Press.

Horner, J., and Fedor, K. H. (1983). Minor hemisphere mediation in aphasia treatment. In: H. Winitz (ed.), *Treating Language Disorders: For Clinicians by Clinicians*. Baltimore: University Park Press.

Huang, M., and Byrne, B. (1978). Cognitive style and lateral eye movements. *British Journal of Psychology*, **69**, 85–90.

Hughes, M-A., and Sussman, H. M. (1983). An assessment of cerebral dominance in language-disordered children via a time-sharing paradigm. *Brain and Language*, **19**, 48–64.

Humphrey, M. E., and Zangwill, O. L. (1951). Cessation of dreaming after brain injury. *Journal of Neurology, Neurosurgery and Psychiatry*, **14**, 322–325.

Hyman, L. M. (1975). *Phonology: Theory and Analysis*. New York: Holt, Rinehart and Winston.

Ingvar, D. H., and Scwartz, M. S. (1974). Bloodflow patterns induced in the dominant hemisphere by speech and reading. *Brain*, **97**, 273–288.

Jackson, J. H. (1866). Notes on the physiology and pathology of language. In: J. Taylor (ed.), (1958) *Selected Writings of John Hughlings Jackson*: Vol. Two. London: Staples Press.

Jackson, J. H. (1874). On the nature of the duality of the brain. In: J. Taylor (ed.), (1958). *Selected Writings of John Hughlings Jackson*: Vol. Two. London: Staples Press.

Jackson, J. H. (1879). On affections of speech from disease of the brain. In: J. Taylor (ed.), *Selected Writings of John Hughlings Jackson*: Vol. Two. London: Staples Press.

John, G. R. (1982). Multipotentiality: a theory of recovery of function after brain damage. In: J. Orbach (ed.), *Neuropsychology After Lashley*. Hillsdale NJ: Lawrence Erlbaum Assoc.

Johnson, J. P., Sommers, R. K., and Weidner, W. E. (1977). Dichotic ear preference in aphasia. *Journal of Speech and Hearing Research*, **20**, 116–129.

Johnson, P. (1977). Dichotically stimulated ear differences in musicians and non-musicians. *Cortex*, **13**, 385–389.

Johnson, R. C., Bowers, J. K., Gamble, M., Lyons, F. M., Presbrey, T. M., and Vetter, R. R. (1977). Ability to transcribe music and ear superiority for tone sequences. *Cortex*, **13**, 295–299.

Jonas, S. (1982). The thalamus and aphasia, including transcortical aphasia: a review. *Journal of Communication Disorders*, **15**, 31–41.

Kawai, I., and Ohashi, H. (1975). Total speech disturbance and cerebral dominance. *Studia Phonologica*, **9**, 40–44.

Kelly, R. R., and Orton, K. D. (1979). Dichotic perception of word pairs with mixed image values. *Neuropsychologia*, **17**, 363–371.

Kent, R. D. (1984). Brain mechanisms of speech and language with special reference to emotional interactions. In: R. C. Naremore (ed.), *Language Science*. Windsor: NFER–Nelson.

Kent, R. D., and Rosenbek, J. C. (1982). Prosodic disturbances and neurologic lesion. *Brain and Language*, **15**, 259–291.

Kershner, J. R., and Jeng, A. G. R. (1972). Dual functional hemispheric asymmetry in visual perception: effects of ocular dominance and post exposural processes. *Neuropsychologia*, **10**, 437–445.

Kershner, J. R., Thomae, R., and Calloway, R. (1977). Nonverbal fixation control in young children induces a left-field advantage in digit recall. *Neuropsychologia*, **15**, 569–576.

Kertesz, A. (1979). *Aphasia and Associated Disorders*. New York: Grune and Stratton.

Kertesz, A. (ed.) (1983). *Localization in Neuropsychology*. London: Academic Press.

Kertesz, A., and Hooper, P. (1982). Praxis and language: the extent and variety of apraxia in aphasia. *Neuropsychologia*, **20**, 275–286.

Kertesz, A., and McCabe, P. (1977). Recovery patterns and prognosis in aphasia. *Brain*, **100**, 1–18.

Kertesz, A., and Sheppard, A. (1981). The epidemiology of aphasic and cognitive impairment in stroke: age, sex, aphasia type and laterality differences. *Brain*, **104**, 177–128.

Kimura, D. (1961). Cerebral dominance and the perception of verbal stimuli. *Canadian Journal of Psychology*, **15**, 166–171.

Kimura, D. (1964). Left–right differences in the perception of melodies. *Quarterly Journal of Experimental Psychology*, **16**, 355–358.

Kimura, D. (1967). Functional asymmetry of the brain in dichotic listening. *Cortex*, **3**, 163–178.

Kimura, D., and Archibald, Y. (1974). Motor functions of the left hemisphere *Brain*, **97**, 337–350.

Kimura, D., and Dornford, M. (1974). Normal studies on the function of the right hemisphere in vision. In: S. J. Dimond and J. G. Beaumont (eds.), *Hemisphere Function in the Human Brain*. London: Elek Science.

King, F. L., and Kimura, D. (1971). Left-ear superiority in the perception of vocal nonverbal sounds. *Research Bulletin 188*, Department of Psychology, University of Western Ontario.

Kinsbourne, M. (1971). The minor cerebral hemisphere as a source of aphasic speech. *Archives of Neurology*, **25**, 302–306.

Kinsbourne, M. (1972). Eye and hand turning indicates cerebral lateralization. *Science*, **176**, 539–541.

Kinsbourne, M. (1974). Direction of gaze and distribution of cerebral thought processes. *Neuropsychologia*, **12**, 279–281.

Kinsbourne, M., and Cook, J. (1971). Generalized and lateralized effects of concurrent verbalization on a unimanual task. *Quarterly Journal of Experimental Psychology*, **23**, 341–345.

Kinsbourne, M., and Hiscock, M. (1977). Does cerebral dominance develop? In: S. G. Segalowitz and F. A. Gruber (eds.), *Language Development and Neurological Theory*. New York: Academic Press.

Kinsbourne, M., and McMurray, J. (1975). The effect of cerebral dominance on time sharing between speaking and tapping by preschool children. *Child Development*, **46**, 240–242.

Kinsbourne, M., and Warrington, E. (1962). A variety of reading disability associated with right hemisphere lesions. *Neurosurgery and Psychiatry*, **25**, 339–344.

Klingman, K. L., and Sussman, H. M. (1983). Hemisphericity in aphasic language recovery. *Journal of Speech and Hearing Research*, **26**, 249–256.

Knox, C., and Kimura, D. (1970). Cerebral processing of nonverbal sounds in boys and girls. *Neuropsychologia*, **8**, 227–237.

Kocel, K., Galin, D., Ornstein, R., and Merrin, R. (1972). Lateral eye movements and cognitive mode. *Psychonomic Science*, **27**, 223–224.

Kohn, B. (1980). Right-hemisphere speech representation and comprehension of syntax after left cerebral injury. *Brain and Language*, **9**, 350–361.

Kornhuber, H. H. (1977). A reconsideration of the cortical and subcortical mechanisms involved in speech and aphasia. In: J. E. Desmedt (ed.), *Language and Hemispheric Specialization in Man: Cerebral ERP's*. Base 1: Karger.

Krashen, S. D. (1972). Language and the left hemisphere. *UCLA Working Papers in Phonetics*, **24**, 1–72.

Lake, D. A., and Bryden, M. P. (1976). Handedness and sex differences in hemispheric asymmetry. *Brain and Language*, **3**, 266–282.

Lambert, A. T. (1982). Right hemisphere language processing II: evidence from normal subjects. *Current Psychological Reviews*, **2**, 139–151.

Lambert, A. T., and Beaumont, J. G. (1982). On Kelly and Orton's 'Dichotic perception of word pairs with mixed image values'. *Neuropsychologia*, **20**, 209–210.

Lamendella, J. T. (1977). The limbic system in human communication. In: H. Whitaker and H. A. Whitaker (eds.), *Studies in Neurolinguistics*, Vol. III. London: Academic Press.

Landis, T., Cummings, J. L., and Benson, D. F. (1980). Le passage de la dominance du langage a l'hemisphere droit: une interpretation de la recuperation tardive lors d'aphasies globales. *Revue Medica de la Suisse Romande*, **100**, 171–177.

Landis, T., Regard, M. Graves, R., and Goodglass, H. (1983). Semantic paralexia: a release of right hemispheric function from left hemisphere inhibition. *Neuropsychologia*, **21**, 359–364.

LaPointe, L. L., and Horner, J. (1981). Pallilalia: a descriptive study of pathological reiterative utterances. *Journal of Speech and Hearing Disorders*, **46**, 90–105.

Larsen, B., Skinhoj, E., and Lassen, N. (1978). Variations in regional cortical blood flow in the right and left hemispheres during automatic speech. *Brain*, **101**, 193–209.

Lashley, K. S. (1929). *Brain Mechanisms and Intelligence*. Chicago: University of Chicago Press.

Lassen, N. A., Ingvar, D. H., and Skinhoj, E. (1978). Brain function and blood flow. *Scientific American*, **239**, 50–59.

Latham, C. (1849). Case of injury to the head followed by a loss of the musical faculty. *Lancet*, **i**, 668–669.

Laurence, S., and Stein, D. G. (1978). Recovery after brain damage and the concept of localization of function. In: S. Finger (ed.), *Recovery from Brain Damage*. New York: Plenum.

Lebrun, Y. (1983). Cerebral dominance for language: a neurolinguistic approach. *Folia Phoneatrica*, **35**, 13–39.

Lebrun, Y., and Lebrun, N. (1971). On the role of visual feedback in writing. *ITL*, **13**, 59–62.

Lebrun, Y., and Rubio, S. (1972). Reduplications et omissions graphiques cher des patients atteints d'une lesion hemispherique droite. *Neuropsychologia*, **10**, 249–251.

Leehey, S., and Cahn, A. (1979) Lateral asymmetries in the recognition of words, familiar faces and unfamiliar faces. *Neuropsychologia*, **17**, 619–635.

Lenneberg, E. (1967). *The Biological Foundations of Language*. New York: John Wiley.

Lesser, R. (1974). Verbal comprehension in aphasia: an English version of three Italian tests. *Cortex*, **10**, 247–263.

Lesser, R. (1976). Lexical–semantic impairment after right-hemisphere damage? Presented at European Brain and Behaviour Workshop, London.

Le Vere, T. E. (1975). Neural stability, sparing, and behavioural recovery following brain damage. *Psychological Review*, **82**, 344–358.

Le Vere, T. E. (1980). Recovery of function after brain damage: a theory of the behavioural deficit. *Physiological Psychology*, **8**, 297–308.

Levin, H. S. (1981). Aphasia in closed head injuries. In: M. T. Sarno (ed.), *Acquired Aphasia*. London: Academic Press.

Levine, D. N., and Mohr, J. P. (1979). Language after bilateral cerebral infarctions: role of the minor hemisphere in speech. *Neurology*, **29**, 927–938.

Levy, J. (1969). Possible basis for the evolution of lateral specialization of the human brain. *Nature*, **224**, 614–615.

Levy, J. (1974). Psychobiological implications of bilateral asymmetry. In: S. J. Dimond and J. G. Beaumont (eds.), *Hemisphere Function in the Human Brain*. London: Elek Science.

Levy, J. (1983). Language, cognition and the right hemisphere: a response to Gazzaniga. *American Psychologist*, **38**, 538–541.

Levy, J., Nebes, R. D., and Sperry, R. W. (1971). Expressive language in the surgically separated minor hemisphere. *Cortex*, **7**, 49–58.

Levy, J., and Trevarthen, C. (1973). Hemispheric specialization tested by simultaneous rivalry for mental associations. Unpublished Manuscript. University of Pennsylvania.

Levy, J., and Trevarthen, C. (1977). Perceptual, semantic and phonetic aspects of elementary language processes in split-brain patients. *Brain*, **100**, 105–118.

Ley, R. G., and Bryden, M. P. (1979). Hemispheric differences in recognizing faces and emotions. *Brain and Language*, **7**, 127–138.

Ley, R. G., and Bryden, M. P. (1981). Consciousness, emotion, and the right hemisphere. In: G. Underwood and R. Stevens (eds.), *Aspects of Consciousness*, Volume II: *Structural Issues*. London: Academic Press.

Liberman, A. M., Cooper, F. S., Shankweiler, D., and Studdert-Kennedy, M. (1967). Perception of the speech code. *Psychological Review*, **74**, 431–461.

Luria, A. R. (1963). *Restoration of Function After Brain Injury*. New York: Macmillan.

Luria, A. R. (1970). *Traumatic Aphasia*. The Hague: Mouton.

Luria, A. R., Naydin, V. L., Tsvetkova, L. S., and Vinarskaya, E. N. (1969). Restoration of higher cortical functions following local brain damage. In: P. J. Vinken and G. W. Bruyn (eds.), *Handbook of Clinical Neurology*, Vol. 3. Amsterdam: North-Holland.

Marcie, P. (1983). Writing disorders associated with focal cortical lesions. In: M. Martlew (ed.), *The Psychology of Written Language*. Chichester: Wiley.

Marcel, A. J., and Patterson, K. (1979). Word recognition and production: reciprocity in clinical and normal research. In: J. Requin (ed.), *Attention and Performance*, Volume 7. Hillsdale, New Jersey: Laurence Erlbaum.

Marr, D. (1980). Visual information processing: the structure and creation of visual representations. *Philosophical Transactions of the Royal Society, London*, **B290**, 199–218.

Marshall, J. C. (1973). Some problems and paradoxes associated with recent accounts of hemispheric specialization. *Neuropsychologia*, **11**, 463–470.

Marshall, J. C. (1977). Disorders in the expression of language. In: J. Morton and J. C. Marshall (eds.), *Psycholinguistics Series—1: Developmental and Pathological*. London: Elek Science.

Marshall, J. C. (1983). Hemispheric specialization: what, how and why. *The Behavioural and Brain Sciences*, **4**, 72–73.

Marshall, J. C., and Newcombe, F. (1973). Patterns of paralexia. *Journal of Psycholinguistic Research*, **2**, 175–199.

Marshall, J. C., and Newcombe, F. (1980). The conceptual status of deep dyslexia: an historical perspective. In: M. Coltheart, K. Patterson and J. C. Marshall (eds.), *Deep Dyslexia*. London: Routledge and Kegan Paul.

Marshall, J. C., and Patterson, K. E. (1983). Semantic paralexia and the wrong hemisphere: a note on Landis, Regard, Graves and Goodglass (1983). *Neuropsychologia*, **21**, 425–427.

Mateer, C. A. (1983). Motor and perceptual functions of the left hemisphere and their interaction. In: S. J. Segalowitz (ed.), *Language Functions and Brain Organization*. London: Academic Press.

Mateer, C. A., and Ojemann, G. A. (1983). Thalamic mechanisms in language and memory. In: S. J. Segalowitz (ed.), *Language Functions and Brain Organization*. London: Academic Press.

Mazziotta, J. C., Phelps, M. E., Carson, R. E., and Kuhl, D. E. (1982). Tomographic mapping of the auditory cortex during auditory stimulation. *Neurology*, **32**, 921–937.

McFarland, K., McFarland, M., Bain, J., and Ashton, R. (1978). Ear differences of abstract and concrete word recognition. *Neuropsychologia*, **16**, 555–561.

McGlone, J. (1977). Sex differences in cerebral organization of verbal functions in patients with unilateral brain lesions. *Brain*, **100**, 755–793.

McGlone, J. (1978). Sex differences in functional brain asymmetry. *Cortex*, **14**, 122–128.

McGlone, J. (1983). Sex differences in human brain organization: a critical survey. *The Behavioural and Brain Sciences*, **3**, 215–227.

McKeever, W. F., and Hulings, M. D. (1971a). Bilateral tachistoscopic word recognition as a function of hemisphere stimulated and interhemispheric transfer time. *Neuropsychologia*, **9**, 281–288.

McKeever, W. F., and Hulings, M. D. (1971b). Lateral dominance in tachistoscopic word recognition performance obtained with simultaneous bilateral input. *Neuropsychologia*, **9**, 15–20.

McKeever, W. F., Larrabee, G. J., Sullivan, K. F., Johnson, H. J., Ferguson, S., and Rayport M. (1981). Unimanual tactile anomia consequent to corpus callosotomy: reduction of anomic defect under hypnosis. *Neuropsychologia*, **19**, 179–190.

McKeever, W. F., Suberi, M., and Van DeVenter, A. D. (1972). Fixation control in tachistoscopic studies of laterality effects: comments and data relevant to Hines' experiment. *Cortex*, 473–479.

Messorli, P., Tissot, A., and Rodriguez, J. (1976). Recovery from aphasia: some factors of prognosis. In: Y. Lebrun and R. Hoops (eds.), *Recovery in Aphasia*. Amsterdam: Swets and Zeitlinger, BV.

Metter, E. J., Wasterlain, C. S., Kuhl, D. E., Hanson, W. K., and Phelps, M. E. (1981).

18FDG positron emission computed tomography in a study of aphasia. *Annals of Neurology*, **10**, 173–183.

Miceli, G., Caltagirone, C., Gainotti, G., and Payer-Rigo, P. (1978). Discrimination of voice versus place contrasts in aphasia. *Brain and Language*, **6**, 47–51.

Miceli, G., Gainotti, G., Caltagirone, C., and Masullo, C. (1980). Some aspects of phonological impairment in aphasia. *Brain and Language*, **11**, 159–169.

Millar, J. M., and Whitaker, H. A. (1983). The right hemisphere's contribution to language: a review of the evidence from brain-damaged subjects. In: S. J. Segalowitz (ed.), *Language Functions and Brain Organization*. London: Academic Press.

Miller, E. (1984). *Recovery and Management of Neuropsychological Impairments*. Chichester: John Wiley.

Milner, B. (1967). Discussion following Rossi and Rosadini 'Experimental analysis of cerebral dominance'. In: C. H. Millikan and F. L. Darley (eds.), *Brain Mechanisms Underlying Speech and Language*. New York: Grune and Stratton.

Milner, B. (1974). Hemispheric specialization: scope and limits. In: F. O. Schmidt and F. Worden (eds.), *The Neurosciences*, Vol III. Cambridge, Massachusetts: MIT Press.

Milner, B., Branch, C., and Rasmussen, T. (1966). Evidence for bilateral speech representation in some non-right-handers. *Transactions of the American Neurological Association*, **91**, 306–308.

Milner, B., Branch, C., and Rasmussen, T. (1968). Observations on cerebral dominance. In: R. C. Oldfield and J. C. Marshall (eds.), *Language: Selected Readings*. Harmondsworth: Penguin.

Milner, B., and Taylor, L. B. (1970). Somesthetic thresholds after commissural section in man. Paper presented at the Meeting of the American Academy of Neurology. Miami, Florida.

Milner, B., Taylor, L., and Sperry, R. (1968). Lateralized suppression of dichotically presented digits after commissural section in man. *Science*, **161**, 184–186.

Mohr, J. P. (1973). Rapid amelioration of motor aphasia. *Archives of Neurology*, **28**, 77–82.

Mohr, J. P. (1976). Broca's area and Broca's aphasia. In: H. Whitaker and H. A. Whitaker (eds.), *Studies in Neurolinguistics*, Vol. 1. New York: Academic Press.

Mohr, J. P., Pessin, M. S., Finkelstein, S., Funkenstein, H. H., Duncan, G. W., and Davis, K. R. (1978). Broca aphasia: pathologic and clinical. *Neurology*, **28**, 311–324.

Monrad-Krohn, G. H. (1947). Dysprosody or altered 'melody of language'. *Brain*, **70**, 405–415.

Monrad-Krohn, G. H. (1963). The third element of speech, prosody and its disorders. In: H. Halpern (ed.), *Problems of Dynamic Neurology*. Jerusalem: Hebrew University.

Moore, W. H. (1974). The right cerebral hemisphere: its role in linguistic processing in aphasia. Unpublished Ph.D. Thesis, Kent State University.

Moore, W. H. (1984). The role of right hemispheric information processing strategies in language recovery in aphasia: an electroencephalographic investigation of hemispheric alpha asymmetries in normal and aphasic subjects. *Cortex*, **20**, 193–205.

Moore, W. H., and Weidner, W. E. (1974). Bilateral tachistoscopic word perception in aphasic and normal subjects. *Perceptual and Motor Sills*. **39**, 1003–1011.

Moore, W. H., and Weidner, W. E. (1975). Dichotic word-perception of aphasic and normal subjects. *Perceptual and Motor Skills*, **40**, 379–386.

Morrow, L., Vrtunski, P. B., Kim, Y., and Boller, F. (1981). Arousal responses to emotional stimuli and laterality of lesion. *Neuropsychologia*, **19**, 65–71.

Moscovitch, M. (1972). A choice reaction time study assessing the verbal behaviour of the minor hemisphere in normal, adult humans. *Journal of Comparative and Physiological Psychology*, **80**, 66–74.

188

Moscovitch, M. (1973). Language and the cerebral hemispheres: reaction-time studies and their implications for models of cerebral dominance. In: P. Pliner, L. Krames, and T. Alloway (eds.), *Communication and Affect: Language and Thought*. New York: Academic Press.

Moscovitch, M. (1976). On the representation of language in the right hemisphere of right-handed people. *Brain and Language*, **3**, 47–71.

Moscovitch, M., and Olds, J. (1982). Asymmetries in spontaneous facial expression and their possible relation to hemispheric specialization. *Neuropsychologia*, **20**, 71–81.

Munk, H. (1881). *Ueber die funktionen der Grosshirnrinde. Gesammelte Mitteilungen aus den Jahren 1880–1887*. Berlin: August Hirshwald.

Myers, P. (1980). Visual imagery in aphasia treatment: a new look. In: R. H. Brookshire (ed.), *Clinical Aphasiology Conference Proceedings*. BRK Publishers, Minneapolis.

Naeser, M. A. (1983). CT scan lesion size and lesion locus in cortical and subcortical aphasias. In: A. Kertesz (ed.), *Localization in Neuropsychology*. London: Academic Press.

Naeser, M. A., and Hayward, R. W. (1978). Correlation between CT scan findings and the Boston Diagnostic Aphasia Exam. *Neurology*, **28**, 545–551.

Naeser, M. A., Hayward, R. W., Laughlin, S., and Zatz, L. M. (1981). Quantitative CT scan studies in aphasia. Part I. Infarct size and CT numbers. *Brain and Language*, **12**, 140–164.

Natale, M., Gur, R. E., and Gur, R. C. (1983). Hemispheric asymmetries in processing emotional expressions. *Neuropsychologia*, **21**, 555–565.

Niccum, N., Rubens, A. B., and Speaks, C. (1981). Effects of stimulus material on the dichotic listening performance of aphasic patients. *Journal of Speech and Hearing Research*, **24**, 526–534.

Nielsen, J. M. (1946). *Agnosia, Apraxia, Aphasia: Their Value in Cerebral Localization*. New York: Hoeber.

Niessl Von Mayendorff, E. (1911). *Die aphasischea symptome und ihre kortikale lokalisation*. Leipzig: Barth.

Nootebohm, F. (1983). Does hemispheric specialization of function reflect the needs of an executive side? *The Behavioral and Brain Sciences*, **4**, 75.

Oakley, D. A. (ed.) (1985). *Brain and Mind*. London: Methuen.

Obler, L. K., Albert, M. L., Goodglass, H., and Benson, D. F. (1978). Aphasia type and aging. *Brain and Language*, **6**, 318–322.

Ojemann, G. A. (1976). Subcortical language mechanisms. In: H. Whitaker and H. A. Whitaker (eds.), *Studies in Neurolinguistics*, Vol. 1. London: Academic Press.

Ojemann, G. A. (1983). Brain organization for language from the perspective of electrical stimulation mapping. *The Behavioral and Brain Sciences*, **2**, 189–230.

Olesen, J., Paulson, O. B., and Lassen, N. A. (1971). Regional cerebral bloodflow in man determined by the initial slope of the clearance of intra-artrially injected 133Xe. *Stroke*, **2**, 519.

Oscar-Berman, M., Rehbein, L., Porfert, A., and Goodglass, H. (1978). Dichhaptic hand-order effects with verbal and nonverbal tactile stimulation. *Brain and Language*, **6**, 323–333.

Oscar-Berman, M., Zurif, E. B., and Blumstein, S. (1975). Effects of unilateral brain damage on the processing of speech sounds. *Brain and Language*, **2**, 345–355.

Paivio, A. (1971). *Imagery and Verbal Processing*. New York: Holt.

Paivio, A., and Ernest, C. (1971). Imagery ability and visual perception of verbal and nonverbal stimuli. *Perception and Psychophysics*, **10**, 429–432.

Patterson, K., and Besner, D. (1984). Is the right hemisphere literate? *Cognitive Neuropsychology*, **1**, 315–341.

Patterson, K., and Bradshaw, J. L. (1975). Differential hemispheric mediation of nonverbal visual stimuli. *Journal of Experimental Psychology*, **1**, 246–252.

Patterson, K. and Kay, J. (1982). Letter-by-letter reading: psychological descriptions of a neurological syndrome. *Quarterly Journal of Experimental Psychology*, **34A**, 411–422.

Penfield, W., and Jaspers, H (1954). *Epilepsy and the Functional Anatomy of the Human Brain*. Boston: Little, Brown.

Penfield, W., and Perot, P. (1963). The brain's record of auditory and visual experience. *Brain*, **86**, 595–696.

Penfield, W., and Roberts, L. (1959). *Speech and Brain Mechanisms*. Princeton: Princeton University Press.

Perecman, E. (ed.) (1983). *Cognitive Processing in the Right Hemisphere*. London: Academic Press.

Pettit, J. M., and Noll, J. D. (1979). Cerebral dominance in aphasia recovery. *Brain and Language*, **7**, 191–200.

Phelps, M. E., Kuhl, D. E., and Mazziotta, J. C. (1980). Tomographic mappings of the metabolic changes in the visual cortex during visual stimulation of volunteers and patients with visual defects. *Journal of Nuclear Medicine*, **21**, 21 (abstract).

Piazza, D. M. (1977). Cerebral lateralization in young children as measured by dichotic listening and finger tapping tasks. *Neuropsychologia*, **15**, 417–425.

Pieniadz, J. M., Naeser, M. A., Koff, E., and Levine, H. L. (1983). CT scan cerebral hemispheric asymmetry measurements in stroke cases with global aphasia: atypical asymmetries associated with improved recovery. *Cortex*, **19**, 371–391.

Popper, K. R., and Eccles, J. C. (1977). *The Self and Its Brain*. Berlin: Springer-Verlag.

Powell, G. E. (1981). *Brain Function Therapy*. Aldershot: Gower.

Premack, D. (1971). Language in chimpanzee? *Science*, **172**, 808–822.

Prins, R., Snow, C., and Wagenaar, E. (1978). Recovery from aphasia: spontaneous speech versus language comprehension. *Brain and Language*, **6**, 192–211.

Prutting, C. (1982). Pragmatics as social competence. *Journal of Speech and Hearing Disorders*, **47**, 123–134.

Puccetti, R. (1973). Brain bisection and personal identity. *British Journal of Philosophy of Science*, **24**, 339–355.

Rabinowicz, B. and Moscovitch, M. (1984). Right hemisphere literacy: a critique of some recent approaches. *Cognitive Neuropsychology*, **1**, 343–350.

Rasmussen, T., and Milner, B. (1977). The role of early left-brain injury in determining lateralization of cerebral speech functions. *Annals of the New York Academy of Sciences*, **299**, 355–369.

Reuter-Lorenz, P., and Davidson, R. J. (1981). Differential contributions of the cerebral hemispheres to the perception of happy and sad faces. *Neuropsychologia*, **19**, 609–613.

Reuter-Lorenz, P., Givis, R., and Moscovitch, M. (1983). Hemispheric specialization and the perception of emotion: evidence from right-handers and from inverted and non-inverted left-handers. *Neuropsychologia*, **21**, 687–692.

Richardson, J. T. E. (1975). Further evidence of the effect of word imageability in dyslexia. *Quarterly Journal of Experimental Psychology*, **27**, 445–449.

Rinn, W. E. (1984). The neuropsychology of facial expression: a review of the neurological and psychological mechanisms for producing facial expressions. *Psychological Bulletin*, **95**, 52–77.

Robinson, R. S., and Benson, D. F. (1981). Depression in aphasic patients: frequency, severity, and clinical–pathological correlations. *Brain and Language*, **14**, 282–289.

Rosner, B. S. (1970). Brain functions. *Annual Review of Psychology*, **21**, 555–594.

Rosner, B. S. (1974). Recovery of function and localization of function in historical

190

perspective. In: D. G. Stein, J. J. Rosen, and N. Butters (eds.), *Plasticity and Recovery of Function in the Central Nervous System*. New York: Academic Press.

Ross, E. D. (1981). The aprosodias. Functional–anatomic organization of the effective components of language in the right hemisphere. *Archives of Neurology (Chicago)*, **38**, 561–569.

Ross, E. D. (1983). Right hemisphere lesions in disorders of affective language. In: A. Kertesz (ed.), *Localization in Neuropsychology*. London; Academic Press.

Ross, E. D., and Mesulam, M-M. (1979). Dominant language functions of the right hemisphere? Prosody and emotional gesturing. *Archives of Neurology*, **36**, 144–148.

Rossi, G. F., and Rosadini, G. (1967). Experimental analysis of cerebral dominance in man. In: C. H. Millikan and F. L. Darley (eds.), *Brain Mechanisms Underlying Speech and Language*. New York: Grune and Stratton.

Sackheim, H. A., and Gur, R. C. (1978). Lateral asymmetry in intensity of emotional expression. *Neuropsychologia*, **16**, 473–481.

Sackheim, H. A., and Gur, R. C. (1983). Facial asymmetry and the communication of emotion. In: T. S. Cacioppo and R. E. Petts (eds.), *Social Psychophysiology*. New York. Guilford Press.

Sackheim, H. A., Gur, R. C., and Saucy, M. C. (1978). Emotions are expressed more intensely on the left side of the face. *Science*, **202**, 434–436.

Sackheim, H. A., Weiman, A. L., and Forman, B. D. (1984). Asymmetry of the face at rest: size, area and emotional expression. *Cortex*, **20**, 165–178.

Saffran, E. M., Bogyo, L. C., Schwartz, M. F., and Marin, O. S. M. (1980). Does deep dyslexia reflect right-hemisphere reading? In: M. Coltheart, K. Patterson, and J. C. Marshall (eds.), *Deep Dyslexia*. London: Routledge and Kegan Paul.

St James-Roberts, I. (1979). Neurological plasticity, recovery from brain insult and child development. *Advances in Child Development and Behaviour*, **14**, 253–319.

St James-Roberts, I. (1981). A reinterpretation of hemispherectomy data without functional plasticity of brain. *Brain and Language*, **13**, 31–53.

Sand, P. L., and Taylor, N. (1973). Handedness: evaluation of binominal distribution hypothesis in children and adults. *Perceptual and Motor Skills*, **36**, 1343–1346.

Sasanuma, S. (1980). Acquired dyslexia in Japanese: clinical features and underlying mechanisms. In: M. Coltheart, K. Patterson, and J. C. Marshall (eds.), *Deep Dyslexia*. London: Routledge and Kegan Paul.

Sasanuma, S., Itoh, M., Mori, K., and Kobayashi, Y. (1977). Tachistoscopic recognition of kana and kanji words. *Neuropsychologia*, **15**, 547–553.

Satz, P. (1980). Incidence of aphasia in left-handers: a test of some hypothetical models of cerebral speech organization. In: J. Herron (ed.), *Neuropsychology of Left Handedness*. New York: Academic Press.

Satz, P., Aschenback, K., Pattishall, E., and Fennell, E. (1965). Order of report, ear, asymmetry, and handedness in dichotic listening. *Cortex*, **1**, 377–396.

Satz, P., and Bullard-Bates, C. (1981). Acquired aphasia in children. In: M. T. Sarno (ed.), *Acquired Aphasia*. New York: Academic Press.

Saya, M. (1979). Blissymbolics: an alternative system of communication for the non-verbal aphasic patient. Paper presented at Canadian Speech and Hearing Conference.

Schmuller, J., and Goodman, R. (1979). Bilateral tachistoscopic perception, handedness and laterality. *Brain and Language*, **8**, 81–91.

Schuell, H., Jenkins, J., and Jimenez-Pabon, E. (1964). *Aphasia in Adults*. New York: Harper and Row.

Schulhoff, C., and Goodglass, H. (1969). Dichotic listening, side of brain injury and cerebral dominance. *Neuropsychologia*, **7**, 149–160.

Schwartz, G., Davidson, R., and Maer, F. (1975). Right hemisphere lateralization for emotion in the human brain: interaction with cognition. *Science*, **190**, 286–288.

Searleman, A. (1977). A review of right hemisphere linguistic capabilities. *Psychological Bulletin*, **84**, 503–528.

Searleman, A. (1980). Subject variables and cerebral organization for language. *Cortex*, **16**, 239–254.

Segalowitz, S. J., and Bryden, M. P. (1983). Individual differences in hemispheric representation of language. In: S. J. Segalowitz (ed.), *Language Functions and Brain Organization*. London: Academic Press.

Segalowitz, S. J., and Stewart, C. (1979). Left and right lateralization for letter matching: strategy and sex differences. *Neuropsychologia*, **17**, 521–525.

Semmes, J. (1968). Hemispheric specialization: a possible clue to mechanism. *Neuropsychologia*, **6**, 11–26.

Sersfetinides, E. A., and Falconer, M. A. (1963). Speech disturbances in temporal lobe seizures: a study in 100 epileptic patients submitted to anterior temporal lobectomy. *Brain*, **86**, 333–346.

Shai, A., Goodglass, H., and Barton, M. (1972). Recognition of tachistoscopically presented verbal and non-verbal material after unilateral cerebral damage. *Neuropsychologia*, **10**, 185–191.

Shanks, J., and Ryan, W. (1976). A comparison of aphasic and non-brain-injured adults on a dichotic CV-syllable listening task. *Cortex*, **12**, 100–112.

Shankweiler, D., and Studdert-Kennedy, M. (1967). Identification of consonants and vowels presented to left and right ears. *Quarterly Journal of Psychology*, **19**, 59–63.

Shapiro, B., and Danly, M. (1985). The role of the right hemisphere in the control of speech prosody in propositional and affective contexts. *Brain and Language*, **25**, 19–36.

Shapiro, A. K., Shapiro, E., and Wayne, H. (1972). Birth, developmental, and family histories and demographic information in Tourette's syndrome. *Journal of Nervous and Mental Disease*, **155**, 335–344.

Sidtis, J. J., Volpe, B. T., Wilson, D. H., Rayport, M., and Gazzaniga, M. S. (1981). Variability in right hemisphere language functions: evidence for a continuum of generative capacity. *Journal of Neuroscience*, **1**, 323–331.

Simirnitskaya, E. G. (1974). On two forms of writing deficit following focal brain lesions. In: S. J. Dimond and J. G. Beaumont (eds.), *Hemispheric Function in the Human Brain*. London: Elek Science.

Skinhoj, E., and Larsen, B. (1980). The pattern of cortical activation during speech and listening in normals and different types of aphasic patients as revealed by regional cerebral blood flow (rCBF). In: M. T. Sarno and O. Hook (eds.), *Aphasia: Assessment and Treatment*. New York: Masson Publishing.

Smith, A. (1966). Speech and other functions after left (dominant) hemispherectomy. *Journal of Neurology, Neurosurgery and Psychiatry*, **29**, 467–471.

Smith, A., and Burkland, C. W. (1966). Dominant hemispherectomy. *Science*, **153**, 1280–1282.

Sparks, R. (1981). Melodic intonation therapy. In: R. Chapey (ed.), *Language Intervention Strategies in Adult Aphasia*. Baltimore: Williams and Wilkins.

Sparks, R., and Geschwind, N. (1968). Dichotic listening in man after section of neocortical commissures. *Cortex*, **4**, 3–16.

Sparks, R., Goodglass, H., and Nickel, B. (1970). Ipsilateral versus contralateral extinction in dichotic listening resulting from hemispheric lesions. *Cortex*, **6**, 249–260.

Sparks, R., Helm, N., and Albert, M. (1974). Aphasia rehabilitation resulting from melodic intonation therapy. *Cortex*, **10**, 303–316.

Sparks, R. W., and Holland, A. L. (1976). Method: melodic intonation therapy for aphasia. *Journal of Speech and Hearing Disorders*, **41**, 287–297.

Speaks, C., Carney, E., Niccum, N., and Johnson, C. (1981). Stimulus dominance in dichotic listening. *Journal of Speech and Hearing Research*, **24**, 430–437.

Sperry, R. W. (1961). Cerebral organization and behaviour. *Science*, **133**, 1749–1757.

Sperry, R. W. (1964). The great cerebral commissure. *Scientific American*, January, 42–52.

Sperry, R. W. (1974). Lateral specialization in the surgically separated hemispheres. In: F. O. Schmidt and F. Worden (eds.), *The Neurosciences*, Vol. III. Cambridge, Massachusetts, MIT Press.

Sperry, R. (1984). Consciousness, personal identity and the divided brain. *Neuropsychologia*, **22**, 661–673.

Sperry, R. W., and Gazzaniga, M. S. (1967). Language following surgical disconnection of the hemispheres. In: C. H. Millikan and F. L. Darley (eds.), *Brain Mechanisms Underlying Speech and Language*. New York: Grune and Stratton.

Sperry, R. W., Gazzaniga, M. S., and Bogen, J. E. (1969). Interhemispheric relationships: the neocortical commissures. Syndromes of hemispheric disconnection. In: P. J. Vinken and G. Grugn (eds.), *Handbook of Clinical Neurology*. Amsterdam: North Holland.

Strausse, E., and Moscovitch, M. (1981). Perception of facial expressions. *Brain and Language*, **13**, 308–322.

Studdert-Kennedy, M., and Shankweiler, D. (1970). Hemispheric specialization for speech perception. *Journal of the Acoustical Society of America*, **48**, 579–594.

Studdert-Kennedy, M., Shankweiler, D., and Pisoni, D. B. (1972). Auditory and phonetic processing in speech perception. Evidence from a dichotic study. *Cognitive Psychology*, **3**, 455–466.

Suberi, M., and McKeever, W. F. (1977). Differential right hemispheric memory storage of emotional and non-emotional faces. *Neuropsychologia*, **15**, 757–768.

Subirana, H. (1958). The prognosis in aphasia in relation to the function of cerebral dominance and handedness. *Brain*, **8**, 415–425.

Sussman, H. M. (1982). Contrastive patterns of interhemispheric interference to verbal and spatial concurrent tasks in right-handed, left-handed and stuttering populations. *Neuropsychologia*, **20**, 675–684.

Sweet, R. D., Solomon, G., Wayne, H., Shapiro, E., and Shapiro, A. (1973). Neurological features of Gilles de la Tourette's syndrome. *Journal of Neurology, Neurosurgery and Psychiatry*, **36**, 1–9.

Tallal, P., and Newcombe, F. (1978). Impairment of auditory perception and language comprehension in dysphasia. *Brain and Language*, **5**, 13–24.

Taylor, J. (ed.) (1958). *Selected Writings of John Hughlings Jackson*: Vol. II. London: Staples Press.

Taylor-Sarno, M. (1969). *The Functional Communication Profile*. New York: New York University Medical Center.

Tikofsky, R. S., Kooi, K. A., and Thames, M. H. (1960). Electroencephalographic findings and recovery from aphasia. *Neurology*, **10**, 154–156.

Tucker, D. M. (1981). Lateral brain function, emotion, and conceptualization. *Psychological Bulletin*, **89**, 19–46.

Tucker, D. M., Roth, R. S., Arneson, B. A., and Buckingham, V. (1977). Right hemisphere activation during stress. *Neuropsychologia*, **15**, 697–700.

Tucker, D. M., Watson, R. G., and Heilman, K. M. (1976). Affective discrimination and evocation in patients with right parietal disease. *Neurology*, **26**, 354.

Tueber, H-L. (1974). Why two brains? In: F. O. Schmitt and F. G. Warden (eds.), *The Neurosciences Third Study Program*, Cambridge, Massachusetts: MIT Press.

Tzeng, O. J. L., Hung, D., and Cotton, B. (1979). Visual lateralization effect in reading Chinese characters. *Nature*, **282**, 499–501.

Van Lancker, D. (1972). Language processing in the brain. UCLA Working Papers in Phonetics, **23**, 22–31.

Van Lancker, D. (1975). Heterogeneity in language and speech. UCLA Working Papers in Ponetics, **29**.

Van Lancker, D., and Fromkin, V. A. (1973). Hemispheric specialization for pitch and 'tone'; evidence from Thai. *Journal of Phonetics*, 1, 101–109.

Vignolo, L. (1964). Evolution of aphasia and language rehabilitation: A retrospective exploratory study. *Cortex*, 1, 344–367.

Von Monokow, C. V. (1911). Lokalization der Hirnfunktionen. *Journal fur Psychologie und Neurologie*, 17, 185–200.

Von Monokow, C. (1969). Diaschisis. Excerpt translated from the German by G. Harris. In: K. H. Pribram (ed.), *Brain and Behaviour 1: Moods, States and Mind*. Harmondsworth: Penguin.

Wada, J. (1949). A new method for the determination of the side of cerebral speech dominance. A preliminary report on the intracarotid injection of sodium amytal in man. *Medical Biology*, 14, 221.

Walsh, K. W. (1978). *Neuropsychology: A Clinical Approach*. Edinburgh: Churchill-Livingstone.

Wapner, W., Hamby, S., and Gardner, H. (1981). The role of the right hemisphere in the apprehension of complex linguistic materials. *Brain and Language*, 14, 15–33.

Warrington, E. (1981). Concrete word dyslexia. *British Journal of Psychology*, 72, 175–196.

Wechsler, A. F. (1973). The effect of organic brain disease on recall of emotionally charged versus neutral narrative text. *Neurology*, 23, 130–135.

Weigl, E., and Bierwisch, M. (1970). Neuropsychology and linguistics: topics of common research. *Foundations of Language*, 6, 1–18.

Weinreich, V. (1969). Problems in the analysis of idioms. In: J. Puhvel (ed.), *Substance and Structure of Language*. Los Angeles: University of California Press.

Weinstein, E. A., and Kahn, R. L. (1955). *Denial of Illness: Symbolic and Physiological Aspects*. Springfield, Illinois: Charles C. Thomas.

Weiss, M. J., and House, A. S. (1973). Perception of dichotically presented vowels. *Journal of the Acoustical Society of America*, 38, 583–589.

Wernicke, C. (1874). *Der aphasische Symptomencomplex*. Breslau: Max Cohn & Weigert.

West, J. F. (1978). Heightening the action imagery of materials used in aphasia treatment. In: R. H. Brookshire (ed.), *Clinical Aphasiology Conference Proceedings*. Minneapolis: BRK Publishers.

West, J. F. (1983). Heightening visual imagery: a new approach to aphasia therapy. In: E. Perecman (ed.), *Cognitive Processing in the Right Hemisphere*. New York: Academic Press.

Wexler, B. (1980). Cerebral laterality and psychiatry. *The American Journal of Psychiatry*, 137, 279–291.

White, M. J. (1969). Laterality differences in perception: a review. *Psychological Bulletin*, 72, 387–405.

Wigan, A. L. (1844). *The Duality of the Mind*. London: Longman.

Wilson, D. H., Reeves, A., and Gazzaniga, M. S. (1978). Division of the corpus callosum for uncontrollable epilepsy. *Neurology (NY)*, 28, 649–653.

Wilson, D. H., Reeves, A. G., Gazzaniga, M. S. and Culver, C. (1977). Cerebral commissurotomy for the control of intractable seizures. *Neurology*, 27, 708–715.

Witelson, S. F. (1974). Hemispheric specialization for linguistic and non-linguistic tactual perception using a dichotomous stimulation technique. *Cortex*, 10, 3–17.

Yamadori, A., Osumi, Y., Masuhara, S., and Okubo, M. (1977). Preservation of singing in Broca's aphasia. *Journal of Neurology, Neurosurgery and Psychiatry*, 40, 221–224.

Yamaguchi, F., Meyer, J. S., Sakai, F., and Yamamoto, M. (1980). Case reports of three dysphasic patients to illustrate rCBF responses during behavioral activation. *Brain and Language*, 9, 145–148.

Yeni-Komshian, G. H., and Gordon, J. F. (1974). The effects of memory load on the right ear advantage in dichotic listening. *Brain and Language*, **1**, 375–381.

Yund, E. W., and Efron, R. (1975). Dichotic competition of simultaneous tone bursts of different frequency II. Suppression and ear dominance functions. *Neuropsychologia*, **13**, 137–150.

Young, A. W. (ed.) (1983). *Functions of the Right Hemisphere*. London: Academic Press.

Young, A. W., and Ratcliff, G. (1983). Visuospatial abilities of the right hemisphere. In: A. W. Young (ed.), *Functions of the Right Cerebral Hemisphere*. London: Academic Press.

Zaidel, E. (1975). A technique for presenting lateralized visual input with prolonged exposure. *Vision Research*, **15**, 282–289.

Zaidel, E. (1976). Auditory vocabulary of the right hemisphere following brain bisection and hemidecortication. *Cortex*, **12**, 191–211.

Zaidel, E. (1977). Unilateral auditory comprehension on the Token Test following cerebral commissurotomy and hemispherectomy. *Neuropsychologia*, **15**, 1–10.

Zaidel, E. (1978a). Auditory language comprehension in the right hemisphere following cerebral commissurotomy and hemispherectomy: a comparison with child language and aphasia. In: A. Caramazza and E. B. Zurif (eds.), *Language Acquisition and Language Breakdown*. Baltimore: Johns Hopkins University Press.

Zaidel, E. (1978b). Lexical organization in the right hemisphere. In: P. A. Buser and A. Rougeul-Buser (eds.), *Cerebral Correlates of Conscious Experience*. Amsterdam: Elsevier/North Holland Press.

Zaidel, E. (1982). Reading by the right hemisphere: an aphasiological perspective. In: Y. Zotterman (ed.), *Dyslexia: Neuronal, Cognitive and Linguistic Aspects*. Oxford: Pergamon Press.

Zaidel, E. (1983). A response to Gazzaniga: Language in the right hemisphere, convergent perspectives. *American Psychologist*, **38**, 542–546.

Zaidel, E., and Schweiger, A. (1984). On wrong hypotheses about the right hemisphere: commentary on K. Patterson and D. Besner, 'Is the right hemisphere literate?' *Cognitive Neuropsychology*, **1**, 351–364.

Zangwill, O. (1960). *Cerebral Dominance and Its Relation to Psychological Function*. Edinburgh: Oliver and Boyd.

Zangwill, O. (1967). Speech and the minor hemisphere. *Acta Neurol. Psychiatr. Belg.*, **67**, 1013–1020.

Zollinger, R. (1935). Removal of left cerebral hemisphere: report of a case. *Archives of Neurology and Psychiatry*, **34**, 10055–1064.

Zurif, E. B. (1974). Auditory lateralization: prosodic and syntactic factors. *Brain and Language*, **1**, 391–404.

AUTHOR INDEX

SUBJECT INDEX